# It's Only Hair

hair loss help and humor

By

Christine Mager Wevik

Copyright © 2010 by Christine Mager Wevik

Cover and interior design by Masha Shubin | Inkwater.com

© 2010 Dmitri Mihhailov. Image from iStockPhoto.com
Author photo by Sandy Photography

ISBN: 979-8-9863920-2-8

HAIR (FROM "HAIR")
Music by GALT MacDERMOT Words by JAMES RADO and GEROME RAGNI
©1966, 1967, 1968, 1970 (Renewed) JAMES RADO, GEROME RAGNI,
GALT MACDERMOT, NAT SHAPIRO and EMI U CATALOG All Rights Administered by EMI U CATALOG {Publishing} and ALFRED PUBLISHING CO., INC. (Print)
All Rights Reserved      Used by Permission

All rights reserved. No part of this book may be reproduced or transmitted in any form or by any means whatsoever, including photocopying, recording or by any information storage and retrieval system, without written permission from the publisher and/or author.

# Dedication

I owe a deep and never-ending gratitude to those who always believed I could do whatever I set my mind to, no matter how outrageous it seemed: first of all to my children, my sisters and brothers, my parents-in-law, but most of all, my dearest friends. To my Brenda, the greatest "twin" sister and friend that a girl could ever have - I'll forever mourn the day we stopped holding hands just because it looked dumb. To my friend and neighbor and almost sister, Ann – you are patience, gentleness, and kindness personified and a constant inspiration. To Joanne – you are far too kind and generous for your own good – don't ever change because I learn so much from you. To Ginger – I want to be you when I grow up. You are fearless and strong, and I admire you so much. And finally to my best friend, my husband, and love of my life, Doug – you have given me the opportunity and motivation to know and love myself better. Thank you for your patience, your continued support, and for loving me "anyway."

# Acknowledgements

Thank you to The National Alopecia Areata Foundation for their help in providing information about alopecia for me, my book, and millions of Alopecians throughout the world. Their commitment to encourage and fund research to find a cause and ultimate cure for alopecia, to support those with the disease, and to raise public awareness is awe inspiring.

Thank you to my dermatologist, Dr. Gene Burrish, of Sanford Dermatology, Sioux Falls, SD. He has been exceedingly patient with me and all my endless questions.

Thank you to my family doctor, Dr. Scott Ecklund of Sanford Clinic Family Medicine, in Sioux Falls, SD. Never mind about my hair - he knew what was more important: the rest of me.

And finally, thank you to all who shared their own personal stories of hair loss so that I could better understand the wide range of emotions felt by all who lose their hair, and how very important it is to be understood and accepted, no matter what our differences are.

*But the Lord said to Samuel, "Do not look on his appearance or on the height of his stature, because I have rejected him; for the Lord does not see as mortals see; they look on the outward appearance, but the Lord looks on the heart."*

*1 Samuel 16:7*


*"If you love something, let it go. If it comes back, it's yours. If it doesn't, it never was."*

*Author unknown*


*"Don't worry! Be happy!"*

*Bobby McFerrin*

# Table of Contents

Dedication .................................................................... iii

Acknowledgements............................................................ v

Preface ........................................................................ xiii

Introduction ................................................................ xvii

Chapter One: "Inquiring Minds Want to Know".............. 1
   *Questions and answers about living with hair loss and its causes.*

Chapter Two: Just the Facts, Please. ................................... 5
   *Just plain facts about alopecia.*

Chapter Three: White Tape and Other Miracle Cures ..... 12
   *Real and imagined treatments and cures for hair loss.*

Chapter Four: The Journey .............................................. 19
   *Chemo: Friend and foe.*
       Chemo, The Monster .............................................. 20

"Angela" .................................................................. 25
"Barbara" ................................................................ 28
"Gina" ..................................................................... 29
"Margaret" .............................................................. 31

**Chapter Five: Touché, Toupée!** ........................................ 34
*Take that, androgenetica!*

**Chapter Six: "Little Shavers"** ........................................... 42
*Little people with big challenges.*

"Brad" ..................................................................... 47
"Colin" .................................................................... 48
Colin's mother, Nichole ........................................... 49

**Chapter Seven: Alopecians Anonymous** ......................... 52
*Experiences with alopecia.*

"My name is Chris, and I'm an Alopecian." ............... 52
"Lexie" .................................................................... 72
On Men and Alopecia ............................................. 80
"Bob" ...................................................................... 81

**Chapter Eight: The Naked Truth** ..................................... 83
*Options for hair-challenged people.*

WIGS: ..................................................................... 84
HATS: ..................................................................... 91
AU NATUREL: ........................................................ 94
MAKEUP! ............................................................... 98

**Chapter Nine: Seeking Insurance Coverage for Cranial Prostheses** ......................................................... 102
*Getting insurance companies to cover full cranial prostheses.*

**Chapter Ten: "Hair"** ........................................................ 105
*A Cowsills song devoted to, you got it, Hair.*

Big Hairy Deal or The Great "Love-of-Hair" ............ 107

Chapter Eleven: God Speaks............................................ 117
　　*Spirituality and preserving our inner spirit.*

Chapter Twelve: It's All in Your Head ........................... 135
　　*Attitude: Thinking, then acting.*

Epilogue: "A House of a Different Color"....................... 152

Resources ...................................................................... 157

# Preface

Perhaps I should begin by addressing the title of this book, as it does need some defending. I am not, by any means, trying to minimize anyone's loss. It is a question and it is also a statement. It may even be an attitude. How one interprets the title depends entirely on his or her state of mind.

When I wrote the original preface for this book, my statements, and thereby my attitude, was a much angrier one. But a lot of things have changed since then. I have learned much through the course of this disorder, and throughout my life. One thing that I learned was that "No one can make you feel inferior without your permission." Eleanor Roosevelt said that. It's so true. Secondly, I learned that humor and a little tougher skin can get us through a lot. So with that in mind, I would like to share a story that my sister, Brenda, shared with me (author unknown):

There was a woman who woke up one day, and in getting ready for her day, looked into her mirror and discovered that she had only three hairs left on her head. She stared into the mirror for a long while. Finally, she said to herself, "Today, I think I will wear a braid!" So she put her three hairs into one braid and went on her way.

The next day, the woman woke up, and in getting ready for her day, looked into her mirror and discovered that she had only two hairs left on her head. She stared into the mirror for a long while. Finally, she said to herself, "I think, today, that I shall wear pigtails!" So she put her two hairs into two pigtails and went on her way.

The next day, the woman awoke, went to her mirror, and discovered that she had only one hair left on her head. She stared into the mirror for a long while. Finally, she said to herself, "Today, I will wear a ponytail!" So she put her one hair into a ponytail and went on her way.

The next day, the woman awoke, went directly to her mirror, and saw that she had no hairs left on her head. No hairs left at all. She stared into the mirror for a long while. Finally she said to herself, "Hurray!!! Today I don't have to fix my hair!!"

I know that hair loss is difficult to deal with. I also

know that it's not the end of the world. So if what I think, that attitude can literally make us or break us, is true, doesn't it behoove us to choose happiness?

When I said that a lot has changed I think the most important thing was me. I changed. I choose not to be victimized or minimized by my hair loss. I choose happiness. I choose me.

# Introduction

*In the beginning, God created hair. It's function: protection. It provideth a shield from the hot sun to keep us cool, and in the cold, a warm cap to crown us. And God said "This is good."*

Hair was, of course, also a convenient toga for Eve, the first to discover nudity. (Or was that Adam?) As time went on, and I beg for your mercy on my chronological mayhem, it is speculated that in cavemen days the mane was used in the barbaric practice of dragging a mate from cave to cave, after the usually mating ritual of clubbing the intended on the head. Hair, by now, was becoming a nuisance, getting matted, bug-infested, and caught on every object possible, like tree branches where the idea for the noose was patented, and under rocks, thereby creating the idea for area rugs.

And then, on one fateful day, rather than leave the

entangled person there to die as usual, onlookers gather their courage, pooled their intelligence, and decided, after much deliberation and animated arguing, to cut the hair. Wielding sharp bones and rocks, they set to work. Surprisingly enough, the cutting did not cause pain. The hapless victim was freed.

The rescue party stared in stony silence at "The Different One." They looked at each other. Tension was mounting. Was "The Different One" to be a social outcast forevermore? Should they stone him to death and put him out of his misery? Dare they gather him under their collective wings and hide him deep in a cave until he becomes normal again? *Would* he ever be normal again?!

Someone in the crowd cleared his throat and tentatively braved the comment, "Me like it!"

After several sighs of relief, smiles, and slaps on the back, the first beauty salon was founded, and thus began the never-ending journey into the fashion world of hair.

It's Only Hair

Chapter One

# "Inquiring Minds Want to Know"

Questions and answers about living with hair loss and its causes.

**Q. What is alopecia?**
A. It's a mysterious disease that causes baldness. (See Ch. 2)

**Q. What causes it?**
A. No one knows. It seems to be an autoimmune disorder, where the body mistakenly fights off hair like an allergy. (See Ch. 2)

**Q. Is it contagious?**
A. No, but it *can* be replicated.

**Q. Is it hereditary?**
A. Not exclusively, but heredity sometimes plays a role. People with alopecia usually have someone in their family who had it, or some other autoimmune disorder, such as hay fever, asthma, etc. (See Ch. 2)

**Q. Are there different types of alopecia?**
A. Yes. There is Alopecia Areata, (patchy baldness,) Alopecia Totalis, (hair loss on the head,) and Alopecia Universalis, (hair loss of the entire body). There are also very rare forms of alopecia that involve scarring of the scalp, causing permanent hair loss.

**Q. Can it affect other parts of the body?**
A. Yes, alopecia can affect any hair bearing sight on the body. It can also cause stippling of the nails. (See Ch. 2)

**Q. Can alopecia make me sick, affect my health in other ways?**
A. No. Although baldness can make people *appear* ill, alopecia does not affect the health of the body in any other way than to cause hair loss. Most Alopecians are healthy in every other respect.

**Q. Is it caused by nerves?**
A. No. So relax and maybe your hair will grow back. (See Ch. 2)

**Q. Is Chapter 2 the only chapter in this book?**
A. No. It's just the most boring so I need to push it a little bit more.

**Q. Can the hair ever grow back?**
A. Certainly. The hair follicles are undamaged by alopecia and often it grows back without treatment. But if this is not the case, there are treatments that may work

to encourage hair growth until this condition turns itself off. (See Ch. 3)

**Q. Is there a cure for alopecia?**
A. No. If there was, there would be no reason for this book, so I'm hoping they hold off on a cure until after publication. Seriously, though, there is no cure for alopecia, and the causes are still unknown as well. But there are treatments that may work to encourage hair growth until this condition turns itself off. Didn't I just say that? How many times do I have to tell you: See Ch. 3.

**Q. How is alopecia different from male pattern baldness?**
A. Androgenetica, male and female pattern baldness and thinning, is hereditary, and it does involve damage to the hair follicle. Take heart, though. There are some drugs that can stimulate hair growth, with varied results, for this type of baldness also.

**Q. What about hair loss from chemotherapy treatments? Is it permanent?**
A. No.

**Q. Why does the hair fall out from chemo treatments?**
A. The drugs given to kill cancer cells in the body also damage the hair follicle cells. Once the drugs are discontinued, the hair follicle cells begin to do their job again.

**Q. I'm self conscious about not having hair. What should I do?**
A. Everything you did before you lost your hair, but do it with confidence! You are still special, with or without hair! (See all chapters)

**Q. Should I avoid any activities or events that may cause my hair piece to come off?**
A. Absolutely not! The only things one needs to avoid while wearing a wig or hair piece are open flames and low hanging branches.

**Q. What should I say if someone asks me if my hair is "real"?**
A. Say, "Can you see it?" When they say, "Yes," tell them, "Then I guess it's real!" But remember to smile!

**Q. What should I say if someone asks me if it's "mine"?**
A. Tell them, "Yes, and I have the receipt to prove it."

**Q. Will being bald always be this painful?**
A. No. With support from family and friends, counseling, information, and a sense of humor, you will overcome the trauma of your loss. Remember that this is a loss like any other and you have the right to grieve. But eventually, you will move on to acceptance, and with acceptance comes happiness.

Chapter Two

# Just the Facts, Please.

Just plain facts about alopecia.

The definition of alopecia in any given dictionary is "Baldness." (Thanks. That's a big help.) And in some dictionaries that choose to elaborate, it also means "mange in foxes." (Great. Now I'm a mutt with an embarrassing condition.)

Clinically, alopecia has a more definitive description. Alopecia Areata is a common (all my neighbors have it) condition that results in hair loss on the head or any hair-bearing site, such as a beard. Hair loss usually starts with a few small, round, smooth spots. In many cases, the hair grows back within a few months, even without treatment. But also in many cases, the condition returns or worse, spreads until all the hair on the head is gone which is called Alopecia Totalis, and hair loss on the entire body is called Alopecia Universalis. More than two million people in this country have some form of alopecia. There are also some who experience other effects related to alopecia, like stippling (pin-hole appearance) of the nails. And there are some rare forms of alopecia which can cause scarring.

Fortunately, except in the case of scarring alopecia, the hair follicle remains alive and alert, sitting there drumming it's little follicle fingers, waiting for the go-ahead to grow hair, contrary to popular belief that the head is dead, never to grow hair again. So don't give up hope, kids. We just have to wait for a cure. And doctors and scientists researching alopecia believe they are very close to finding the answers to the mysteries of alopecia.

Another condition that can cause sudden hair loss is called telogen effluvium, which is a condition in which the hair moves through its growth cycle very fast, then falls out. It tends to affect new mothers, people who may be on low protein diets, suffer from very high fevers, or have an adverse reaction to drugs. This condition is usually temporary, resolving itself eventually without treatment.

In alopecia, the hair follicle slows down the production of hair and becomes very small. Normal, functioning hair follicles on the scalp produce 0.35 mm of hair each day. Whatever degree of hair loss is present, the hair follicle is alive and there is the possibility of regrowth. Some patients respond well to treatment, of which there are many, with as many degrees of success. As of yet, there are no cures for alopecia, only treatments, which are covered further in a separate chapter. There are some rare forms of alopecia that cause scarring of the skin, which in turn, causes permanent damage, and therefore, permanent hair loss. In any case, aside from the hair loss, and in some, stippling of the nails and minor skin changes, Alopecians are otherwise healthy.

Alopecia occurs in both males and females of all ages, but occurs most often in young persons. According to my dermatologist, Dr. Gene Burrish at Sanford Dermatology in Sioux Falls, SD, the younger the patient with alopecia, the more severe it is likely to be. And, as in my case, if regrowth occurs, the chances of reoccurrence of alopecia are greater.

Being the unpredictable disease that it is, alopecia can turn itself on, causing hair loss, and off again, allowing hair to grow. What triggers this condition to start and stop? No one knows. Doctors do not know what causes alopecia to develop in our system, but theorize that many factors may play a role in causing the condition to erupt or surface, tripping hair follicles into a dormant phase. There are treatments that, for some, may prod the hair follicle to function normally, and the hair begins to grow on its own without continued treatment. But with many treatments that work, once the treatment is halted, so is the growth, and, unable to stay in a growing phase, the hair follicle goes dormant again and hair loss occurs. Continued and permanent hair growth depends solely on whether the condition turns itself off. Until recently, doctors thought stress played an important role in the cause of alopecia. And Gramma was certain of this, too. "It's nerves. Relax! Don't be so nervous!" (Oh, if I had a nickel for every time I heard that...) I'm sure stress was largely responsible for *triggering* the condition in my body, causing hair loss, because my hair loss occurred during very stressful times in my life. But, not unlike my cold sores that occur occasionally, alopecia is always in my system, and any shock to my system such as an illness, severe changes in diet, stress, etc. can bring it on. So, in short, stress does not *cause* alopecia. If that were the case, I would fit right in with 90% of the adult population. ALL lawyers and doctors would be bald. And teachers. And parents. And air traffic controllers. Anyway, as I was saying, 90% of adult population……

Doctors theorize that any stress to the immune system can flip that nasty little switch to "ON." These stressors could be anxiety, crash diets, hormonal changes, thyroid disorders; whatever lowers the defense in the immune system. Some doctors even suggest that changes in seasons (less sunlight) or environment (climate: humidity, temperature, sunlight, precipitation, etc.) may affect our immune systems. Who knows- it may be triggered by a change in one's own phone number.

While alopecia is not considered to be exclusively hereditary, those who have relatives with alopecia are more likely to be afflicted. In one out of five alopecia patients, someone in his or her family has also had it. Alopecia often occurs in families whose members may have had hay fever, asthma, atopic eczema or other autoimmune conditions such as vitiligo, thyroid disease, pernicious anemia, or Addison's disease. (Forgive my cynicism, but doesn't everyone have a relative, distant or not, that has ONE of these afflictions?) It is now common speculation that alopecia is an autoimmune process (a type of "self-allergy," if you will). The body mistakenly forms antibodies against the hair follicle cells, seeing them as "foreign," and thus, destroys them as a form of "self-defense," (Stupid, STUPID antibodies! My own body is betraying me, rejecting parts of itself, for God's sake! What's next?! My ears?! Maybe someday I'll sneeze and find a SPLEEN in my tissue!) My doctor explained it to me this way: The body thinks the hair follicle cells are foreign, not supposed to be there. So it sends the white blood cells (USUALLY the good guys) to crowd around the hair follicle to fight them off. These (confused, a.k.a. stupid) immune cells secrete a substance which inhibits the hair from growing. (Please stop secreting!)

Some of the doctors and scientists wonder if their research needs to back up and take a different fork in the road. They question whether this truly is an autoimmune disorder, if perhaps alopecia is a condition that lies only in the hair follicle, rather than being a systemic disorder. For example, if one were to transplant a piece of scalp with hair to a person with alopecia, would hair continue to grow on this piece of scalp and not on the rest, or would it lose the hair, or would it spread to areas previously afflicted with alopecia? Research is being done with mice to determine whether alopecia is a disorder of the immune system or of the hair follicle itself. (Can you imagine little bald mice wearing itty bitty mouse wigs and toupees? Isn't the imagination a wonderful, entertaining thing?)

So many theories, so many questions! There is one theory that almost everyone with alopecia questions, but nevertheless believes. A major cause of alopecia:

SIN. Well, folks, there is no scientific evidence to support the belief that alopecia is our punishment for being (God help us) human. So sin away. I was thoroughly convinced that I was bald because I was "bad," or didn't love God enough or couldn't give up Ho-Ho's for lent or SOMETHING. While I am prepared to say that God didn't do this TO me, I am also more than hesitant to believe that God can cure me. To put that much hope and faith into a single, if not last, opportunity for a cure is more than I am emotionally capable. Enough about God for now. He's got a whole chapter of His own.

Whether you have had alopecia for a while or if it's a fairly new and confusing experience for you, you are more than likely going to be asked why you are bald, and what its cause is. There are many people out there with alopecia who, like Ellen Degeneres, are "coming out," and need to know that there are others like them, that there's someone out there that they can relate to, get to know, and give and receive support. You will eventually find a groove in which you feel comfortable. And *if* you choose to be open about your baldness, you can create an "approachable aura" about you. Smile confidently! Talk freely and positively! Initiate conversations! It can even *make you* feel better *if you* weren't feeling so sprite. I don't mind being asked. I find it very uplifting to know that I can help someone who may be going through the same things I have gone through. I've come to the realization or revelation, if you will, that all most people want out of life is to know that they've made a difference in the world, that they've left a legacy; and helping someone, making a difference to even one person, can be that legacy. So I tell them. And answer their questions. I have alopecia. I've had it for 29 years. Yes, completely bald. No, they don't know what causes it. No, there is no cure. Yes, there are many treatments. No problem. Here's my name and number if you (your friend, daughter, cousin, ...) want to call.

Of course, sometimes I just want to be a stinker. I'd like to go au naturel' and when someone asks me why I'm bald, what's the cause, I'd simply like to say, with furtive glances and maybe a wink, "I'm Alopecian." Those familiar with alopecia will know what I mean. Those who aren't will make their own assumptions. To Alopecians, who could be anyone without hair for whatever reason, its meaning is clear. We belong to an elite membership of intelligent, fun, creative, resilient bald individuals. To non-Alopecians, it could mean any number of things. It could mean I'm alien, (from the country of Alopecia, or to those with an overexcited imagination, from the planet Alopecia.) It could imply a political or moral stance, (I'm against exploitation of flowers), a religious belief, (I worship mushrooms, domes of all kinds), a medical condition, (such as,"I'm dyslexic"), or a statement of sexual orientation, (I'm not touching that one.) And for those who care to inquire further, it's a disease.

Regardless, alopecia is a mystery to doctors and Alopecians alike and while the causes and cures are challenging the doctors, the greatest challenge of all belongs to Alopecians: coping.

Chapter Three

# White Tape and Other Miracle Cures

Real and imagined treatments and cures for hair loss.

Thanks to the National Alopecia Areata Foundation, there is research being done on the possible causes and treatments of alopecia. The NAAF, a non-profit organization, was founded by Ashely Siegel, a woman with alopecia, to help those with alopecia and to help fund research for the disease. Unfortunately, baldness does not rank high on the list of priorities for cures. But there are dedicated doctors and scientists working diligently to unlock the mysteries of alopecia. Depending on which article you read and who wrote it, the cure for alopecia is just out of reach, or not in our lifetime. Personally, I have to maintain the belief that it is just out of reach and in my lifetime. (I hope they hurry 'cuz I don't plan to - or want to - live forever. First of all, I wouldn't get to meet the Big Guy, and I'm not talking about Clint Eastwood, though he's a close second, and secondly, I'd have to learn the metric system.)

# b

Since so little is known about the cause of alopecia, doctors can only speculate on what course of treatment will be effective.

There are many types of treatments that have been found to encourage hair growth in alopecia patients. The most popular form of treatment is cortisone, applied topically or injected into the scalp or eyebrows. Cortisone seems to work by turning off the immune system, and after injections, the lymphocytes seen around the hair ball are decreased. Sometimes, systemic cortisone injections are administered to the patient, usually in the hip, and this shocks the body into growing hair. Systemic cortisone injections, or steroids as they are widely known, are not usually recommended by physicians because of the dangerous side effects, which include palpitations, nausea, etc. And, as with all the other treatments for alopecia, steroids offered only a minimal degree of success - hardly worth the risks involved. I must admit that in my desperation to grow hair I was prepared to take the risk. But my doctor advised against it, stating that, like all other treatments for alopecia, once it is discontinued my hair would probably fall out again. Actually, he stated the risks, and I weighed them: moodiness, "uh-huh...," potential heart problems, "ok....," nausea, "all right...," puffiness and weight gain, "Nope. Huh-uh. Forget it." However, topical cortisone and transdermal cortisone injections have a fairly good success rate. When I had Alopecia Areata, and my hair was falling out in patches, the topical and injections into my scalp worked pretty well. It seemed that I was able to keep up with the disease by treating the spots. Eventually, my hair grew back and all was normal for a couple years or so. Then I'd find a bald spot on my head and I'd fly into a panic and call the doctor, and off we were again, trying to stay ahead of the disease. My doctor noted that I was usually less susceptible to the disease when I was pregnant. But, well aware of the fact that pregnancy usually results in a child, I chose baldness. (I love my four children very much and wouldn't trade them for anything in the world, including a full head of hair, but my body and my sanity wouldn't permit me to bear children for the rest of my life.) (Neither would my husband, for that matter.)

The most recent and most promising discovery in the area of treatments of hair loss is Minoxidil, a drug originally developed to treat hypertension. Patients taking it in tablet form to lower their blood pressure noticed hair growing on their scalps, as well as fuzz also appearing on other parts of their bodies. Researchers found that when Minoxidil (brand name, Rogaine) was applied directly to the scalp that "substantial" hair growth occurred on the scalp after about three months. Minoxidil has about a 30% success rate as a hair growth treatment, and more research is needed to find out how to make Minoxidil more effective. Minoxidil testing was originally done only on men who had substantial hair loss due to male-pattern baldness. However, there is more research being done with Minoxidil on patients with alopecia, including women. At the time Minoxidil's effects became news, it was not recommended for people with hair loss due to alopecia because there was little research done to substantiate claims of hair growth in these patients. It was not recommended by my doctor, either, because of that fact and because the treatment was cost prohibitive, costing $100 dollars a month or more, and, again, hair growth halts when the treatment is discontinued. Further studies of Minoxidil's effects showed that the 5 percent solution, which is approved for use in Canada, has better growth results compared to that of the 2 percent solution approved for use in the United States. Consequently, the companies marketing Minoxidil sought approval from the FDA to sell the 5% solution of Minoxidil in the United States and it is now available over the counter. A fairly new drug seeking competition with Minoxidil's apparent monopoly is finasteride, marketed by Merck as "Propecia," a 1 mg dosage, and "Proscar," a 5 mg dosage. Proscar was approved by the FDA in 1992 for the treatment of enlarged prostate. And, as with Minoxidil, it was found to stimulate hair growth for men. Proscar can be prescribed by a doctor. Propecia has rare side effects, but 1 to 2 percent of those tested did experience sexual difficulties. And Propecia should not be taken by women, or even handled by women because of serious side effects, including birth defects. Propecia was just recently approved in the USA for use in the treatment of hair growth.

    Another treatment in aiding hair growth is anthralin ointment, a tar-like synthetic substance that has been used widely in treating psoriasis. Anthralin ointment is applied once daily and washed off after a few hours, or as little as an hour, depending on the concentration of anthralin. Anthralin treatments work best in patients with mild, patchy alopecia. The drawbacks to using this ointment are that it can be quite irritating, and can cause a temporary brownish discoloration of the skin where applied. Tip: Don't use your good washcloths to scrub this stuff off your head. If it weren't for the skin irritation of anthralin, the tanning bed business would cease to exist.

There is also a drug called DNCB (chloro-dinitro-benzene). This is basically a drug used to irritate the skin on the scalp to cause an allergic rash and attract lymphocytes to the areas where applied. Lymphocytes are a type of white blood cells. White blood cells help fight infections and allergens. (Like hair?!) Doctors studying the effects of DNCB believe that lymphocytes may aid in causing the hair follicles to grow hair. They, the lymphocytes, just mistake the hair for an allergen, and release a substance that inhibits hair growth. They're confused. (*I'm* confused.) Perhaps the reasoning is that if the white blood cells are busy attacking an ACTUAL allergy, they wouldn't be attacking an IMAGINARY allergy. So wouldn't it be smarter to apply this stuff to the bottoms of our feet and get those confused lymphocytes out of our hair? (Maybe they couldn't smell an allergy that far away.) Maybe lymphocytes have their own departments: Head Lymphocytes, (they're the top guys), Facial Lymphocytes, Underarm Lymphocytes, (usually very warm, caring types), General-Body Lymphocytes, (will never make it to the top because they just don't work as hard) and let's not forget about

Pubic Lymphocytes, (they're the guys at the bottom: not respected, ridiculed, labeled as outcasts, but more fun at parties.)

Where were we? Oh, yes. Treatments. And last, but not least, PUVA. PUVA is the combination of the drug Psoralin, a light-sensitizing medication, and the exposure of long wave ultraviolet light, which counteracts in-migrating cells. It's very much like a tanning bed. This requires daily trips to a UVA bed, so this form of treatment, as with all the other treatments, is not only temporary but inconvenient as well. And as with all the treatments, with the exception of Minoxidil, that seem to have varied success rates in causing hair to grow for Alopecians, the overall factor is that they all work to suppress the immune system and its mistaken fight against the hair as an allergen.

And now, to address the chapter's title: White tape and other miracle cures. Gramma Viola, bless her heart, thoroughly believes that there is some magic ingredient in white tape that can actually draw a splinter or sliver to the surface of the skin. So I started thinking: Why not combine this theory with all the other home-remedies I've been offered? There's magnets, worn on top of your head and in your shoes, which are believed to create "a positive flow of the natural balance of magnetism in your body." (m-hm.) Then there's aloe vera, the best all-natural, all-curing, primitive, new-age drug ever discovered. And vitamins, which some swear by and others swear at, and I won't even mention the one about chicken dung. So I'll get up every morning, wipe aloe vera juice all over my head, (forget that chicken dung thing), take my vitamins with more aloe vera juice, apply my magnets and wrap myself in white tape. What do I have to lose, except my dignity, and whatever love Gramma had for me?

Chapter Four

# The Journey
### Chemo: Friend and foe.

I can see my family and friends, smiling and waving, wishing me well. I can see my home, with all its comforts and security, waiting for my return. There is color and beauty and life in front of me. But then Chemo turns me around. I am facing a long, arduous, and painful journey. I see no color, or beauty, and the life I see is full of fear, uncertainty, and misery. Then Chemo tells me, "This is the only way. You must begin your journey now, and keep in mind what awaits you on your return. It will be difficult, and you may lose, but the only way to return to the life you know is to leave it and go on this journey."

I begin with faltering steps. Chemo pushes me ahead whether I'm ready or not. I have gone only a short distance, and I am already weakening when Chemo stops me and says, "I will give you some boots." I thank Chemo and continue again. Then Chemo stops me and says, "But I will take your clothing."

*cmw*

## Chemo, The Monster

Let me begin this chapter by saying that the whole theme of this book deals with the human ego. And compared to the seriousness of a disease such as cancer, the subject of hair loss, alone and of itself, is incredibly petty. However, I felt it necessary to include a large section of the population of Alopecians: Chemo victims. They are indeed victims of the cruel monster, Chemo, but very often the victors in their battle. Chemotherapy, a treatment used to fight many forms of cancer, in many cases, causes its patients to lose their hair. (Your odds of losing your hair during chemo depend on what types of drugs are used in your treatment. Be sure to ask your doctor about which drugs will, will not, or will possibly cause hair loss.) The drugs used in chemotherapy that destroy the cancer cells also damage the hair follicle cells, thus causing them to stop hair production, and eventually the hair falls out. Even though the hair loss is most usually temporary, it is still traumatic and painful.

When I'm not wearing my wig, I am often mistaken for someone going through chemo, which leads me to believe that the vast majority of America believes that this is the only cause of total hair loss. In the course of writing this book, I had the wonderfully enlightening experience of interviewing many people who suffered from hair loss, including those who have gone through, or are going through, chemotherapy. And in my interviews of the later, I was surprised at my embarrassment and shame of the pettiness of my condition while these brave souls fought for their lives.

What was even more surprising to me was learning

that for cancer patients undergoing chemotherapy treatments, losing their hair was by far the most challenging or difficult part of their disease. One could callously assume that these patients place their appearance above life itself. But that's not what they're doing at all. True, they are faced with a life-threatening illness, however, the word "cancer" is not so quickly equated with death as it was 20 years ago. To them, doctors and technology are heroes that will stand up to the challenge and come out on top. They MUST believe that their disease will be beaten before they can even consider engaging in the battle of and for their lives. So much for them to consider:

> Doctors. Technology. Strength. Treatment. Nutrition. Attitude. Hope. Faith. Cures. Miracles. Death does not seem necessarily imminent. Hair loss does.

Chemo patients know that hair loss will be a major sacrifice - a very obvious battle wound for all to see; a red letter proclaiming their indignities suffered in an honorable battle in a not-so-popular war. They know they'll be bald, that their hair will come out a few strands at a time at first, and the loss will escalate quickly, the hair falling out in clumps, littering their pillows, shoulders, and shower drains. They pretend that it won't happen to them. They hope it won't happen to them. Yet they do everything they can to prepare. They stare into the mirror, admiring their hair, imagining their head completely hairless. They order wigs to match their hairstyle. They brush it ever so carefully, they wash it ever so carefully, but then, despite their tenderness and prayers and hopes, they pluck the last of it from the brush, shower drain, and pillow, hopeful no more. The hair loss part of cancer brings the reality of the disease to the foreground, for the patients as well as the public. Many chemo patients describe losing their hair as "adding insult to injury," "a slap in the face."

It's understandable that they should feel this way. Now, not only *are* they sick, they *look* sick. Ask anyone. They'll tell you that bald people look ill. It's common knowledge that when one feels that they look good, they feel good. Even if one chooses to go "topless", there is still the challenge of looking healthy. Makeup, clothing, color, accessories, all of these make a difference. However, when you're throwing up, losing weight, and lack color and energy, that's the least of your concerns. You want to get through the day, period. Eventually, when things ease up and the world beckons you to join in the fun again, you look in the mirror you've tried to avoid, and wonder where to begin.

Begin with realizing that even though you feel shame at your baldness, you have nothing to be ashamed of. Along with the pity that you as a cancer patient have to endure from the public, you should know that there is also unspoken admiration and respect for your determination. Sadly enough, having cancer, going through treatments, losing one's hair is very much like a veteran feeling ashamed of admitting his or her participation in the Vietnam war, wearing the permanent badges of honor: scars, missing limbs, and disabilities. It was duty.

It was necessary. It was difficult, painful, and horrifying. It was a miracle to live through it, and you should be proud. Everyone should be proud.

Pride is not something that is easily acquired. Cancer, like any disease, is a physical occurrence. And even though hair loss is physical as well, its impact is more psychological than physical. It's relatively easy to combat the physical effects of losing hair. Wear a hat. Wear a wig. Wear a scarf. But as secretive as you are, as careful as you are, someone is going to see you bald: *You*. And unfortunately, there is nothing you can wear to hide from yourself. Like I tell those ticks that I find on me after I've been outdoors, "You can run, but you can't hide!"

Without looking at yourself in the mirror, think of how you see yourself. Not your physical self, but your actions, your sense of humor, your kindnesses, your role as mother/friend/wife/sister, the person you *project*. Say a few words and listen to your voice! Sing a little! (Ok, so you don't have to sing.) How do you see yourself? From the inside looking out, you think you're quite all right. And you are. Why should you feel differently about yourself because of what you may see in the mirror? Is that fair to judge upon appearance? It's not acceptable to do it with others, so why do it with yourself? Yes, it's different! It's shocking! It's very bright and shiny! And it's most likely temporary. One reason that hair loss from cancer treatments is so devastating is because the loss is so sudden, abrupt. There is no time to adjust. It's not gradual, spotty, mysterious, or somewhat treatable like it is with Alopecia Areata. It is sudden, total, shocking, and imminent hair loss. It is a disgusting and scary occurrence. Great clumps of the hair that was once cherished is now nothing more than dead tissue, trash. As enamored as you are with hair in general, you may even be repulsed, as I am, to find unattached hair clinging to your hand, hiding in your food, or worst of all, in your mouth. It's not uncommon for people who know they are going to lose their hair to shave their head completely. Losing it can be more painful than not having it. So it's understandable if you are not comforted by the knowledge that chemo hair loss is most often temporary.

As with the other types of hair loss, it's extremely important to like yourself, accept yourself, and when you are challenged, seek help. Support is probably the single most productive therapy one can get when dealing with the challenge of being different. While doctors, therapists, and books may help you analyze *why* you feel the way you do, others who share your plight *show* you the finer qualities of functioning day to day with your malady. They empathize because they are there, where you are. When they say, "I know exactly what you mean!" they mean it.

You may even find yourself fantasizing about or imagining your future hair. And it's not uncommon for hair in chemo patients to return a different color or texture. It's not often that I do this, but at times I find myself planning my future hair. I plan to wear a wig everyday if I notice my hair coming in, and when it's long enough, pull my wig off and surprise everyone. I plan what color I'm going to have it, I plan the hairstyle, I plan to feel it and cherish it. It's not folly. It's hope.

The difference between folly and hope is living for today, but looking forward to tomorrow. I'm not resigning myself to life without hair. I'm committing myself to life itself. Hair is a very small part of the hopes and plans I have for the future. And if the future brings me hair, wonderful. I will be grateful, and then I will get on with it. If not, I will still get on with it.

Don't attach shame to the pain you already have with the disease you are fighting. I sometimes feel shame at people's assumption that I have cancer. I find myself embarrassed that I only suffer from baldness, and I want to tell people that I'm not sick, and yes, I'm thankful it's nothing more serious. I feel petty at even having to explain my illness. Almost like I didn't earn my baldness. Like I got the ribbon without entering the race. There is no shame in being different. Different is what makes us interesting and unique individuals. Wouldn't it be great if everyone thought of recognizing our uniqueness as "celebrating our diversities," rather than prejudging by our differences?

As prevalent as cancer is, there should be no surprise at one more bald person. The lives of those who cross your path may change, but it will most likely be for the better because you are a symbol of strength and courage. And hope. Don't ever forget hope.

## "Angela"

*February 2nd, 1995. FEBRUARY 2ND!!! I will never forget that day as long as I live. I have WHAT? No way!!! The room twirled around me, my head spun, I had a hard time catching my breath. I couldn't at the age of 40 be diagnosed with Cancer!!! That only happens to other people, not me. Well, it doesn't happen only to other people I am proof of that. The next days that followed where a nightmare — diagnosed on Thursday, on Friday, Cat Scan, blood work, x-rays and surgery to implant a port-a-cath for chemotherapy. Saturday was a day to cry and sit numb from all that was happening. Sunday — my first chemotherary — the first of many.*

*I tried to read all I could to prepare myself for the many rounds of chemo, but nothing could prepare me for what was to come. Two weeks to the day of my first chemo, I began to lose my hair. It was a strange day. For the first time since my diagnosis, I felt a strange calm come over me and sleep finally came. I awoke with a strange feeling all over the top of my head It kinda felt like when I was little and my mom would put tight pony tails in my hair and when I took them out I would have what I called "A pony tail itch." I didn't know what to think of it, but about an hour later..... **IT HAPPENED.** My hair began to come out in huge hunks. Crying, I told my husband. With tears in his eyes, he said he understood — but deep down inside I knew no one understood. I didn't want to wash my hair or even comb it. With each swipe of the brush, more and more would come out and I wanted to keep it as long as I could. We had to vacuum my pillow each morning to get all the hair off from the night before. Within about four days, it was gone. Not blotches here and there. GONE. I looked in the mirror and saw someone I had never seen before. I looked naked, ugly, and sick. No matter how I tried I could never look like myself again. Without eyelashes, there was no place to put mascara.*

*Makeup seemed to make me look like a clown. My wig always made me feel like someone else, not Angela. I thought wigs were for movie stars, not someone like me — vomiting, pale, and UGLY.*

*My doctor was wonderful, and would say I looked fine, but I knew he was lying. My friends and family said that my wig looked "so real." No way!! But I accepted their kind words and pretended that all looked fine.*

*It's funny how something like hair can change your attitude about things. I had two choices — laugh and cry. I did a little of both. Before surgery, when things were very uncertain, it was mostly crying. After my surgery, I noticed in the mirror at the hospital, fine peach fuzz was growing on my head. I was so excited, I had to show the nurse. She must have thought I was crazy. You could barely notice it with the naked eye. But it sure made my day a lot better. When it was growing back, I made my family rub my head, so they could feel how much it had grown. At work my wig got caught on a handle and came off in front of a customer; all I could do is laugh and say "bad hair day." You see nothing could ruin my day. I was cancer free and my hair was growing back, what more could a girl ask for?*

*Cancer was scary, but it was also a gift. It has changed my life and I think for the better. I look at a lot of things differently. My compassion for anyone with hair loss has changed because I know first hand the part baldness on your head can play in your attitude towards life.*

*Angela*

## "Barbara"

My name is Barbara. I'm 60. In 1988 I was diagnosed with Paget's disease of the left breast. I had a biopsy and it was malignant, so I had a mastectomy. No cancer in the lymph nodes, so no further treatment. I did elect to have a silicone implant.

Everything was fine until my regular yearly mammogram in October of 1997. It showed a suspicious mass. I had a needle biopsy done and it was malignant. I followed this with a mastectomy of the right breast and also had the silicone implant removed, as I didn't choose to have another implant. Two of the eleven lymph nodes did show cancer, so the doctor recommended chemo. Since we were planning to go to Tucson, Arizona anyway, I chose to have my treatment at the University Medical Center in Tucson. I began my treatment January 5th. (Adrimyicin and cytoxin, very aggressive.) The doctor said, "You will lose your hair in two weeks." Trying to stay positive, I replied, "Oh, maybe I'll be lucky, and I won't." Exactly two weeks later my hair was coming out in handfuls. Nothing can prepare you for the shock. I'd always had easy to manage hair and was always fussy about how it looked.

I would try to brush it and get all the loose hair before I showered. In the shower when I tried to shampoo what was left of my hair it would come out and get stuck between my fingers. I felt angry. Soon, it was all gone and I felt like the cancer was really taking over my life.

My husband and I both have a good sense of humor, which really helps at a stressful time such as this. My husband joked one day when my hair was coming out that if I were a dog or cat, he'd have to put me outside to do my shedding.

Now it was time for hats, scarves, and wigs. I've never liked wearing anything on my head, but that changed. The wigs were hot and uncomfortable as my scalp was very sensitive after the hair loss. I mainly wore a bandana with a black cowgirl hat, which worked well, especially being in the Southwest for four months. I wore that a lot even after my return home to Iowa.

It has now been six months since my last chemo treatment and my hair is only about one and a half inches long. It is a different texture than before. The back came in quite curly and the top is like a "crew cut." I compare it to "indoor/outdoor carpet." I've spent a lot on special shampoos that are supposed to encourage hair growth and scalp treatment. I question if it helps. Sometimes well-meaning friends will say, "Your hair looks fine, you don't need a hat." In my mind, I think, "Would you think the same if it was your hair?"

I hope and pray I remain cancer-free. I go for check-ups every three months. If cancer doesn't "rear its ugly head" again in my life, I guess I will feel the hair loss was worth it, and the least of my worries.

Barbara

## "Gina"

It has been two years since I had chemo and lost all of my hair. I was told from the beginning that the drugs would make me lose my hair. Although, a small part of me thought perhaps it just might not happen to me. I was wrong. Some friends even suggested going and getting my head shaved. I didn't have the strength to do that. I still remember the week of my hair loss clearly. I could tell it was thinning, so I thought maybe if I didn't wash it and combed it ever so carefully it just might not fall out. Wrong. The week of my hair fall-out, it slowly came out in strands at first and then in clumps. I went camping that weekend with my family. I remember being in the campground bathroom and chunks of my hair were coming out. I got some very strange looks from fellow campers. Then, when we got home from camping Sunday night, it was very windy so I remember going on my deck and running my fingers through my hair and letting it blow into the night. That was when I said farewell to my hair, and the next day I started wearing my wig.

Losing hair was like another slap in the face. I was diagnosed with breast cancer and had a mastectomy. First, you have the shock of finding out you have cancer and lose your breast. And, if that isn't enough, you get to lose your hair as well.

People that don't have hair have a sick look. I remember a couple times taking the kids to practice or wherever. I would just have a scarf on, and I could tell they didn't want their friends to see me. I was never one to go bald — I couldn't even do it at home around my family. I always had a bandanna or a scarf on. Even after my hair started coming in, it took me a long time before I gave up my wig.

My most humiliating experience happened in the mall parking lot. It was a very windy day and I was going back to my vehicle. By habit, I always had one hand hanging onto the corner of my wig because it was usually windy, but my hands were full and I let go for a second to unlock the door. Well, my wig flew off and the wind caught it. When I finally got it, I ran back to my vehicle, and had a hysterical cry. It was so humiliating for me, I even started crying telling the story later to my family and co-workers. They thought it was funny. I suppose it was when you think about it, but when it happens to you it's a different story.

At times, I also thought how can I be so vain. Hey, this is just my hair that I'm losing for six months. How do people handle it when it's an illness that is with them on a daily basis. At least I had hope that there would be an end. Or, what would it be like to be disfigured. In that regard, I was very lucky.

As to my hair now, it came back great. It's thick, has more body and is a darker brown. I think back to the easy times of "no hair" when I could just shower, put on my wig and go — no muss, no fuss!

I think I'm a better person now. I've realized what the important things are in life. I think more on a daily basis as I will always have the cancer ghost at my back door, not knowing when and with what force it will strike again.

Gina

## "Margaret"

My doctor warned me almost to the day when it would fall out. He did not refer me for any kind of therapy. In fact, we discussed it very little. I didn't have any options -I needed the treatment to save my life. So... I accepted it as a necessary "side effect" just as I accepted so many other side effects: constipation, lethargy, shortness of breath, peripheral neuropathy, etc., etc., etc.

Hair loss was a significant loss for me. It was a vivid reminder that I had a life threatening disease. Not only did I not feel good physically, now I looked sick, too! There was nothing that compensated for that loss. I have been somewhat self-conscious of my body and careful to keep in shape ... to be *as attractive as I could within the physical constraints (genes) with which I was born.*

As the months passed (4-5) I became less conscious of my baldness, and with the summer months, opted to go without my wig while at home. (I was fortunate to have a well-shaped head.)

My initial reaction was resignation. We shaved my head rather than deal with the hair everywhere. My family was supportive throughout. I know that they preferred my wig in public, though! Especially my (then) 11-year-old son.

While travelling with extended family on a skiing trip, my (then) 4-year-old nephew observed me removing my wig back at the hotel room. He got the most perplexed look on his face, and said, "Aunt Margaret, how did you do that?" I guess I should have checked the room before I traumatized some poor baby!

I don't recall any advice I was given, except maybe to try to get more comfortable without the wig. You know the "Demi Moore" look. Actually, if you removed the bald "stigma," I was quite cute without hair. (A lot of make-up, though.) I couldn't get very comfortable ... although I did go swimming at my high school reunion. (I still looked better than some of my former classmates, if I do say so myself.)

As far as my hair loss' effect on me, I'm more aware of the time, money, and energy we put into hair. The commercials alone were a constant reminder of my awkwardness. I hated that. Spiritually, the effect was little, as I attribute my faith building more to the life-threatening disease than the hair loss.

My first wig was an expensive one: $500. - my knee-jerk reaction to my diagnosis. Matched my color and cut so when the day came, I was prepared with a wig. I ruined that one within a week. (I wasn't cautioned about melting at 250 degrees - or whatever it was.) It melted when I opened the oven to check dinner. My second wig was $60. (I liked it better, too.) My spare was from an American Cancer Society wig bin - free. More expensive wigs aren't necessarily better. Go for fit and comfort, forget about the texture of the hair. How many people actually touch your wig?

I have attempted hair transplants for radiation-induced alopecia. It was a long shot - and proved unsuccessful. (My first round of cancer was treated with radiation resulting in occipital region hair loss: nape of neck and behind ears.)

I can't say there were any painful moments. I was well-cared for. People were sensitive to that loss for me, especially my husband. He highlighted who I was, not what I looked like. Gotta love him....

I have had an attitude change since my hair loss, though. I am certainly more empathetic to others who suffer hair loss. I strive to be less "appearance" conscious (or critical) of others. Most of all, I really appreciate my hair now. I take good care of it. Skip the perms and processing. The classic "you don't know what you've got 'til it's gone."

*Margaret*

Chapter Five

# Touché, Toupée!
### Take that, androgenetica!

While it may be more socially acceptable and definitely more common, male pattern baldness is not without its own difficulties and insecurities. And because it is more common and easily accepted, it is assumed that men don't worry about it or let it bother them. They have no trouble "handling it." They take it in stride. It's no big deal. Many men with receding hairlines, bald spots, and no hair at all would beg to differ.

Why do you suppose men grow their hair 6" longer on one side of their head and comb it over the top of their balding crown? *Can I say just one thing? Comb-overs are* not *convincing!* Why do you suppose that the makers of Minoxidil have a multi-billion dollar business? Why do you suppose there are companies that are getting rich selling hair in a spray can?

Because baldness is painful. For women AND men. And to add insult to injury, men's shining heads are more often the butts of many jokes. Some of those jokers happen to be bald or balding themselves, kind of a "welcome to the club" jab, but for some of the recipients of these comments and jokes, it's no laughing matter. Why is it ok to tease a man about his baldness when you (hopefully) wouldn't DREAM of teasing a bald woman? Because it's inherited? So is cystic fibrosis.

Male-pattern baldness is a hereditary trait that causes men to have thinning of the hair, receding hairlines, and partial or total baldness. This occurs over a number of years, can start as soon as a young man reaches puberty, and can continue into old age. Male pattern baldness is also called androgenetic alopecia because an androgen, a male hormone, is what causes the problem. The main difference between male pattern baldness and alopecia is the functioning of the hair follicle. Researchers believe that in those predisposed to the disease (those who have maternal *or* paternal relatives who have male pattern baldness), the hair follicles start to produce the enzyme 5-alphareductase, which takes hold of the male hormone testosterone from the blood and turns it to dihydrotestosterone, which attacks the hair follicle, weakens it and causes it to shrivel. The hair follicles in male pattern baldness are damaged and therefore less likely to regain the ability to regrow hair, where in alopecia, they are simply dormant, waiting for the signal to begin regrowth.

In women predisposed to hereditary hair loss, it tends to be more diffuse, thinning all over the head, sometimes more so at the hairline or crown, which is not to say that female androgenetica cannot be severe.

There are many who suffer from pronounced, if not profound or total hair loss due to androgenetica. This condition can be especially devastating for women because the hair loss is so frustratingly gradual, but no less noticeable. At what point do they decide that their hair is too thin? At what point do they begin wearing a wig? Since the hair thins all over or predominantly on top, do they wear a wig or a partial? And admittedly, thin hair and bald spots on women are not as common as on men. They are stuck in a permanent state of limbo. Until, of course, all the hair is gone and they are dropped on their back side with little or no promise of regrowth like those with alopecia.

With androgenic alopecia, the hair follicles sustain some permanent damage, but they still have limited ability to regrow hair. In moments of desperation, one with pattern baldness may succumb to the many miracle cures on the market. There are some that claim to "unblock the follicles" thus, allowing the hair to grow. There are some companies that claim hair growth can be found in an all-natural vitamin or herb extract. There are also infomercials on a serum that can regrow hair within an hour, right there on the spot. Some "experts" even claim that hair growth can be induced with a particular shampoo and massage treatment, but many of these treatments are simply "volumizers," which make hair *appear* thicker and fuller. There oughta[1] be a *law!*

Until recently, there has been nothing to substantiate actual claims of hair growth with any treatment except Minoxidil. Some miracles are just accidents realized. Minoxidil was originally taken for hypertension.

(See chapter 3.) Then it was discovered that it caused hair growth. Wah -La! A billion dollars was made! Now, of course, there is Propecia. (Read on).

Male pattern baldness has been of this world long before cures were. And although there still isn't a cure for it, there are treatments. Besides Minoxidil, men have chosen other courses of treatments such as hair transplants, where "plugs" of hair are removed from other hair bearing sights (usually on the head!) and moved to the area where there is balding. This is called grafting, and since hair can only be grafted from the same person it is intended for, once the donor sights become thin, that's it. No more grafting can be done. And transplants almost never eliminate baldness. Another surgical procedure men opt for is called scalp reduction. It involves exactly what the name implies. Surgeons reduce the scalp by removing strips of bald skin and closing up the incision. This procedure is done progressively, at a few thousand dollars each, until the bald area is covered. These reduction procedures can work only if the skin is flexible enough to cover the area that has been removed. As with both of these surgical procedures, the results are not likely to replicate the full head of hair you once had, and there may be some residual scarring, but many have had very satisfactory results. One needs to speak with a professional, such as a dermatologist or plastic surgeon to gather all the facts, and weigh the pros and cons carefully.

For some reason, toupees are funny. Maybe because of all the calamities that involve toupees or "The Rug." All it is is a mini-wig for men. Maybe what seems to be so hilarious is the fact that men can be vain. Maybe it's humorous that men should care about how they look. I don't know, but I fail to see the humor in someone wanting to look their age instead of 20 years older. I don't know what's so funny about a man wanting to look attractive and youthful and healthy. I'll admit that some pretty funny things can happen to people who wear hair pieces. But I'm not so quick to giggle at someone's attempt to feel good about himself.

Not all men are self-conscious about their thinning or receding hair. Some men I interviewed said that they knew they would eventually lose some of their hair, and that it didn't matter much to them. There are women who prefer bald or balding men. "Bald is Beautiful!" It's sexy. It's a sign of virility. And there are many women, like myself, who don't have a particular preference. I don't find bald men unattractive. To me, baldness only signals a lack of hair. Some men said that they didn't like it, but didn't think it was so important that they would spend hundreds of dollars on hair pieces or hair growth treatments. But some men said that they were depressed seeing their hair fall out, self-conscious about their balding pate, and were currently using a hair growth treatment, such as Minoxidil or Propecia, or wearing a hair piece. The numbers seem to be equally divided among these three groups. And then there are those who don't talk about it at all, but seek out alternatives to hair loss or baldness, thereby admitting their insecurities about their looks, or at the very least, are concerned about looking old before their time.

True, baldness doesn't prohibit people from doing

anything they'd like to do, but it can create some challenges in the area of *opportunity* to do anything they'd like to do. One man mentioned to me that when he was being interviewed for jobs, the interviewer mistook him for someone considerably older, and questioned his abilities to perform the tasks involved in the job for which he was applying. That, in itself, seems to be a reasonable justification to wear a hair piece.

I recently watched an infomercial on "hair replacement systems." It was surprising to see the remarkable difference in the men before and after "the process." To say that they all looked "old" before "the process" (as they called it) would be unfair and maybe a little harsh. But I must say that they all looked, well...., younger afterward. Most of these men were prematurely balding for their ages: 24, 29, 19! And I know the main objective of this infomercial was to paint a lovely picture of "how great life is now that I have hair," and to then sell their hair replacement systems. But being of the bald population, I can understand and agree with their assessment of the importance of hair. All the while they're telling how they are more confident, more outgoing, more happy with the way they look, I'm nodding my head, "I know what you mean! Yeah! Yeah!" Here's proof, folks. Here's before, ok. Here's after: Wow! They really did look better: younger, more vital, healthy, *hairy*. This infomercial also contained interviews of passersby at a mall. Most of these passersby were women, and they admitted that, indeed, hair was an important factor in over-all appearance and first impressions. Well, DUH! We all knew that. But we also know that once you love someone, you love them. Period. If hair will make you a more confident, outgoing, happy person, I say, "Go for it!" Make that all-important first impression! Give yourself and the perspective date a chance! Of course, you won't be able to keep your "secret" under your hat forever, but it's a start!

The hair pieces available to men are much the same as those used by women. Men's hair pieces, though, are obviously smaller, unless they are full wigs, and can be integrated into their own hair quite naturally. The challenge associated with men's hair pieces is that, as a rule, men's hair is shorter, and therefore, the hair piece needs to look more natural next to the scalp. In women's hair pieces, the base of the wig can be woven strips of elastic called wefting, camouflaged by kinking and "matting" the hair next to the scalp. This is not so easily done with very short hair on the hair piece. So naturally, men's hair pieces can cost more due to the extra work done to naturalize it.

There are several types of hair pieces available for men and women today. One of the most popular is hair additions. These are vastly popular for people who don't have any type of hair loss, but just prefer a different look now and then. These are pieces of hair, long and short, straight and curly, braided and bunned, that are clipped onto existing hair, or worn on top of existing hair. They can be integrated into the hair with "weaving," a type of fine weaving and braiding to make it adhere to the head. This weaving will last for weeks before it needs to be done again. A hair addition can also be bonded with a type of glue to the existing hair, as well. Some hair pieces are worn over the hair, and the hair is pulled through holes in the hair piece to blend the real with the fake. And then there are complete and partial wigs and hair pieces that are worn on top of bald skin, and attached with wig tape, which can last a couple days, or removed whenever desired.

So, as you see, the choices are many. One just needs to consider how important hair is. Is it important enough to spend hundreds of dollars on hair pieces and medicines? Is it important enough to spend thousands of dollars on surgeries and doctors? It is important if YOU feel it's important. Everyone deserves to feel good about themselves, and YOU are no exception. It is important to feel attractive and acceptable. Hair loss can be devastating, and we all are aware of certain priorities that may come before our hair, but essentially, you must know you are worth whatever investment you can afford, whenever you can afford it. And no one can make that justification or distinction but YOU.

Chapter Six

# "Little Shavers"
### Little people with big challenges.

Seeing a child in pain is probably a parent's worst nightmare. The feelings of helplessness and frustration are overwhelming. Anyone who has ever loved a child knows the protective instincts that surge forth, and without hesitation, would take that child's place to spare them any more suffering. Unfortunately, that is one prayer that is probably heard the most, and granted the least. So in the meantime, those of us who love children also have a responsibility to help them realistically.

I'd like bring up some important points on dealing with hair loss of children and young adults. First of all, talk with children openly about their hair loss, what it is, how they feel, and what their concerns and questions may be. Be honest and direct, but don't elaborate too much. He or she may get the feeling that you think about it, talk about it, and read about it 24 hours a day, and maybe it's a much bigger deal to *you* than to *them,* and maybe they should worry about it more.

Don't pamper them too much, or treat them differently than any of your other children. Each child has his or her own concerns, and we deal with each concern accordingly. But if baldness and its challenges seem to be the greatest concern in your family, everyone will eventually resent the special treatment, including the child who gets all the special treatment.

Before ordering a wig, or taking charge of your child's head, find out how your child feels about it. After all, it *is* happening to your child and not to you. Does he feel it's necessary? Does he bring it up frequently? Have you noticed a marked change in the personality since the his hair loss? Is he having trouble making or meeting new friends? Is he having trouble in his schoolwork? Talk with him. If he seems to be taking a lot of ribbing in school about it, go to the school and talk with the teachers, principal, and maybe even your child's class about why your child doesn't have any hair. Explain that he's not sick, if that is the case, that it's not contagious, and he can do everything everyone else can do. Answer questions. Explain that differences in people just make life more interesting. Some people are short, some are tall, some have different talents in art, gym, math, or English, many people have different colored skin, different colored hair, eyes, etc., but that's great! Ask some of the kids how they differ from one of their friends. I truly believe that as a society we should celebrate the varied and wonderful and fascinating heritage, personality, and talents that make us each unique individuals. Ask your child's teacher about doing a class project about the differences between people. Talk to the school counselor and ask him or her to guide you through the steps I've suggested. They will be happy to help, since it is their primary goal to see that students have support, concern, and involvement from their parents.

Most of all, try to keep in mind that this is happening to your child, not you. Respect his needs, and listen, listen, listen. If you rush right out and buy a wig your child may get the feeling that you are embarrassed of or for him or her. He needs to feel love and acceptance for himself and from you, no matter how he looks. If he feels that maybe he would just like a hat, great! Hats are fun for kids and although many schools throughout the country have dress codes that don't allow hats, your school may make an exception for your child for this situation. And it should be pointed out at the time that the hat could be more for protection than cover up, that your child has nothing to be ashamed of, and you support whatever decision he makes.

Throughout all of your child's experience without hair, he should be getting the message from you, the parent that he's ok the way he is. Should the subject of wigs come up, it should be your child's doing. Unless your child hints about a wig or you sense your child is struggling emotionally and not able to talk openly with you about one, your bringing it up could indicate to the child that his looks or general appearance is a great concern to you. And nothing other than hair will replace hair. Wigs and hats come off, and a child could be more traumatized by this experience than any other experience he could encounter, including the taunting of classmates. Maintain the attitude that you have confidence that your child can do anything he or she sets out to do. Encourage him, support him, and above all, love and accept him the way he is. If you convey in any way to your child or to others that his or her baldness embarrasses you or makes you upset or bitter or angry, your child may emulate your behaviors. In addition to affecting the way your child reacts, it will also affect the way your child feels.

Your child may feel guilty for not fulfilling your expectations of the kind of child he or she feels you wanted, or your child may feel guilty for causing you so much distress, disappointment, sadness, embarrassment, and anger. Seeing these emotions in you may even scare your child, since he looks to you for strength, reassurance, and security. Have you ever flown in an aircraft that was experiencing turbulence or "mechanical difficulties"? If so, then you, like me, have more than likely looked to see the reaction of the flight attendants. Your mind is screaming, "We're going down! We're going down! Brace! Brace!", but when you look at the flight attendants, they're very calmly handing out peanuts, not scrambling to don their life preservers and oxygen masks. (And this is one of those times that you are *so* glad your mouth didn't obey your mind.) Well, it is in this way that your child looks to you. Granted, you will not and cannot always be there to protect and reassure your child in every discouraging or frightening or disturbing situation. But when you are present when a "situation" occurs, remind yourself that you are the captain of your own ship. Take control. Hand out peanuts!! It may not take much of an imagination to picture this: You are shopping with your young child when another child, or maybe even an adult, says something out loud, or whispers and stares. It has probably happened to you. How do you react? It is much easier to take on the hurt and embarrassment, stuff it, and move on. I know this reaction all too well. Confrontation is much more difficult. But it is within your power to give a positive reaction to a negative action. Stay positive. Smile! Call them back. It's not necessary to acknowledge their reaction to your child's condition. Just simply introduce them to your child, saying something like, "This is my son, Danny. He's seven years old. He looks a little different, doesn't he? You know what? He's allergic to his hair and it *just fell out!* But he's perfectly healthy. What are your names? How old are you? We're so glad to meet you. Do you like playing football? So does Danny..." And so on. Not only will your child know that you are proud of him, but he or she will also gain the confidence to face more "situations" in the future, with or without you. Even a wink and a smile will go a long way in alleviating embarrassment at loud, "painfully honest" comments of other children, while their mothers slowly "die." (a deep shade of red.) We all know how children are much more inclined to ask questions when they are curious, like, "What's wrong with that kid?" as well as other thought-compelling questions like, "Where do ants go when it snows?", and, "Do boogers float?" Well, I applaud their forthrightness and curiosity. I, for one, would much rather answer questions directly than to feel the weight of the stares. And, incidentally, boogers do not float.

In some ways, I believe I was fortunate to have gotten alopecia when I was married and in my twenties, and not when I was in junior high or high school. I find myself saying that it could have easily been one of my children who had alopecia and not me, and I'm so thankful that it was me. I know of so many mothers who wish it were them instead of their child. Well, all I can say is give children some credit. They're resilient, honest, innately loving and trusting, and are born with a healthy sense of self-esteem, but they know nothing of who they are that we don't teach them. Perhaps we could all learn a thing or two from these innocent little creatures and their natural ability to adapt.

## "Brad"

*While my family was shopping one day, two 8-year-old boys walked by our 4- year-old, Bobby. They laughed, pointed, and uttered the inevitable classic, "He's got no hair!" Sure, grammar and manners were not these boys' strong suit, but I just get tired of hearing such comments. Bobby, too, was visibly upset by the callous "observation" offered up by two mean, but then again, typical members of today's "Jerry Springer" society. In an effort to soothe Bobby, I offered up a bit of spontaneous, but not well- thought-out fatherly wisdom.*

*"Bobby, it doesn't matter at all that you haven't got any hair." Bobby's response was immediate - keep in mind that*

this kid is FOUR YEARS OLD! "But it matters to THEM!" My heart sank, my throat tightened, and my eyes watered with searing tears of agony.

I was stumped. I had just been outsmarted by my 4-year-old, "my-reason-for- living" son. His comment revealed insight, poignancy, passion, and even a rhythm that was way beyond his years. It was from his heart. At that moment, I knew that there was going to be a new level of emotion just around the corner. Bobby starts kindergarten in September. Our family is going to have to brace ourselves for emotional gymnastics like this everyday. And we've got to do it bravely. Heck, I've got tears rolling down my face just typing this letter.

Brad

# "Colin"
### 9 years old

I will share my story with you. Here is my story. When I had lost my hair I didn't know because I was only nine months old at the time. It was fun growing until kindergarten. The first day when I got on the bus somebody said, "Hello, bald Mr. Clean." I was mad but I ignored him and sat at a seat. I have been teased a lot in my life like at the park and places like that and by my friends before they knew me. It is very fun being bald because you don't have to get hair cuts, shampoo your hair, or condition your hair. Being bald also helps when you are swimming because you don't have to worry about hair getting in your eyes. The only bad thing about being bald is that you get teased a lot everywhere. But once you get to know everybody you don't really get teased a lot unless you meet new people like I did this year in school, their names are Kristen and

Mike. At first they teased me for a couple of weeks and then they realized that they were just hurting my feelings. The rest of my life has been great being bald. I play baseball, football, and I take swimming lessons in the last level. I think it would be fun to be able to play or be pen pals with another bald kid. I guess it is cool being bald.

Sincerely,<br>Colin

## Colin's mother, Nichole

Our nine year old, Colin, began losing his hair when he was ten months old, and he was completely bald by his first birthday. He may have one advantage in that by growing up with no hair, eyelashes, or eyebrows, he does not recollect what it is like to have hair; therefore, he has not experienced the trauma of losing his hair. Of course, that does not mean that we, his parents, have not experienced the pain of watching our son grow up without hair.

Through the years we have helped Colin deal with being called "baldy," "Mr. Clean," and other names. He seems to handle himself pretty well, but I anticipate the real battle will begin in the teenage years.

Last year, the first day of school was one of the worst experiences of anxiety that we have seen him face. He seemed excited as he prepared for school. But as the time to leave approached, he asked me if I would drive him to school rather than having him take the bus. I told him that I preferred that he take the bus, but that I would meet him at school. He proceeded to tell me that he was sick and didn't think he should go. I suggested that he go, and if he continued to feel sick, I would be more than happy to pick him up. That's when his tears started. Colin explained that every year there is a new kid who always seems to pick on him and call him names. It usually starts on the bus and continues through the day until finally the kid tires of it.

That took me by surprise as I thought he had been handling it so well. I explained to him that he could be like this for the rest of his life and need not feel embarrassed or ashamed I told him to be proud - hair or no hair.

He took the bus and I told him that I would meet him in the classroom. I was surprised to see him waiting for me on the school steps. Colin has never been afraid of school. He settled into his classroom, but when I told him I was leaving I was surprised that he asked me to stay. In the past, he had been so excited to see his friends that he didn't even acknowledge me. It broke my heart to leave him, but I felt that the best thing for him to do was to face his fears. Those were a couple of tough weeks. Mom, Dad, and the teachers cannot always be there for a child, and children have to learn to handle their own battles.

We have always treated Colin with the same rules as our daughter. We don't baby him about his alopecia areata. Some times are harder than others, but I truly believe that if I allow him to shy away from the world, that I am doing an injustice by validating his fear that he won't be accepted. I once watched a mother chase her 6-year-old son with Alopecia Areata around a play area to make him put on his hat. It was she who was uncomfortable if he didn't have on a hat. She also did not enroll him in school because she thought it would be devastating for him. This boy had patches that weren't even noticeable unless you were looking for them. The boy did not seem bothered and no one else paid attention to the fact that *he was losing his hair. Most other kids will accept a child with Alopecia Areata, and if there is some teasing and stares, the child with Alopecia Areata will be able to deal with it.*

*Colin has a lot of friends. One of his best friends had no clue what was wrong with Colin until last week when Colin mentioned something about his Alopecia Areata. His friend looked at him and said, "What are you talking about?" Colin explained while his friend listened and then they went right back to playing. (In my conversation with Nichole, she mentioned that there were even children in Colin's school classes that told their mothers they wanted to have a "haircut" just like Colin's!)*

*I would like to offer a word of advice to other parents who are dealing with this: teach your children to be proud of who they are, challenge their fears, and never give them false hopes. When they learn to accept who they are, so will everyone else. The cruelty of the mean children will wear off. Your child will be a stronger person if you allow them to deal with it. Talking to teachers, the principal, and counselors makes a huge difference.*

*Nichole*

Chapter Seven

# Alopecians Anonymous
Experiences with alopecia.

**"My name is Chris, and I'm an Alopecian."**

I can't recall what my reaction was when I was told I had alopecia. I only remember thinking, "Good. There's a name for it. Therefore, there's a cure." (And hand over the prescription, Doc.)

Not so fast, Missy.

I'd never heard of this weird thing called alopecia. But the doctor seemed to refer to it quickly enough; surely he has heard of it, encountered it, cured it. "We-e-e-l-l-l, we don't know what causes it, and we don't know how to cure it." Thank you. I want a refund.

I'm not blaming the doctors for not having a cure. I'm sure that alopecia is next to last on the "Must Find a Cure" list, last being U.T.S. (Ugly Toenail Syndrome); however, that doesn't make it any easier to live with.

My experience with alopecia began in the fall of 1980. I noticed some small, smooth patches of skin on my head. Hmm. That's odd. I wasn't alarmed. But after they began to grow in size, I became concerned. I showed them to my gramma. SHE was alarmed. So I went to the doctor and he diagnosed it as alopecia. He gave me some Halog solution to rub on it 4 times a day. The bare spots continued to grow over the next few months. I lost the hair on my calves. (No big loss.) Gramma became more distraught. She'd wail every time I showed her my bald spots. (I quit doing that.)

Toward late spring, I noticed hair growing back into the bare spots on my head. (The hair never returned to my calves, nor would my calves ever see a *drop* of Halog solution. I thought of it as a fringe benefit of my condition.) Needless to say, I was quite relieved.

About four years later, a few months after the birth of my second child, my condition returned. This time when I went to see my dermatologist, I was not so cavalier and he was not so kind with his prognosis. He told me that some people get alopecia once and it grows back, and that's the end of it. BUT, for someone who has recurring alopecia, the news is not very promising. The alopecia will likely continue to return, until eventually, the hair falls out completely and never comes back. By now, I was panic-stricken. But, it grew back once before. I was determined it would grow back again. And I would *will* it to stay. It did grow back, with cortisone shots, but my will was ineffective when it came to this disease.

Over the next few years, it seemed that my condition would come and go about every two years, starting in the fall, (how appropriate), and lasting until, usually, late spring. The hair loss was more profuse each time, and with each episode, another portion of my body hair would be lost, never to return. I lost the hair on my thighs. Then my forearms. Spreading upward. It was an ominous sign. Up to this point, the hair always returned to my head. And when my hair grew back, it was always just a little bit thinner. I could handle thinner. Then in May of 1993, I went through some particularly stressful times, which I believe contributed to triggering this disease. I lost all the hair on my body, including eyebrows and eyelashes. I was already struggling with depression. This was certainly NOT a good thing.

My opinion of myself was not healthy, or even fair, to begin with. Now I am supposed to deal with *this?* I had everything one could possible hope for - (with the exception of hair) a wonderful, loving, supportive husband, four beautiful, healthy children; a lovely home; security; family; friends; I was depressed.

After much counseling, I realized that my depression was due, in part, to a chemical imbalance, and also low self-esteem, guilt, and anxiety. Growing up in a dysfunctional family, and then marrying someone (my first husband) who fed my insecurities with verbal and emotional abuse, did nothing for my self-esteem. My first act of self-preservation was to divorce my then husband. But one cannot divorce their past. And, not knowing how to face my problems, I stuffed them.

My stuffing continued into my new marriage, and I was full with my past and present problems. Everyday challenges became insurmountable. I was overwhelmed with all the work involved with living. Depression crept into my life. I eventually sought help, first trying various antidepressants, then hospitalization and counseling, more drugs, and finally, electro-convulsive therapy, or ECT's, also commonly known as "shock treatments," along with more counseling. My doctors told me I suffered from PTSD, or Post Traumatic Stress Disorder from a rather ugly incident involving my ex-husband and a sawed-off shotgun.

I believe the ECT's were more effective than any other treatment I received, although the doctors recommended I follow them with more drug therapy. I do not like taking pills. I consider myself a lightweight. Other than over-the-counter pain medications, everything I took made me feel weird. Tired. Irritable. Weak. Generally speaking, I felt it wasn't helping. So I decided to feel better. I felt strong enough to make a conscious effort to "heal thyself." I felt I needed to take a more active part in my mental health, rather than expecting everyone else to "fix" me. It was, after all, MY life, and I had to live it, and no one would know how to do that, or be able to do that, but me. So, I give myself much credit for my mental health. I worked as hard as anyone and I didn't even get paid. (At least not monetarily!)

It was during my hospitalization for depression in 1993 that my hair fell out for the last time and never returned. And while I think I am coping quite well with my baldness, there's not a day that goes by that I don't miss my hair, think about my hair, hope and pray for hair, or curse this wicked disease. Is that coping? Well, if I'm still alive, and enjoying the process of living, that's all the criteria I need to meet to qualify as "coping." And I can honestly say that if there suddenly appeared a "Cures for All Ailments" line, and "for a limited time only," I'm sure I could step aside and allow every other ailment to take my place .....except for that person with the ugly toenails. After years of living without hair, and encountering dozens of people with hair loss of varying degrees and varying reactions to it, I realize that coping to one person can be completely different than coping to another. I know women who are completely bald and have no compunctions about wearing absolutely nothing on their head when they go out in public. And I, on the other hand, can't bring myself to do that. Then again, I am not bothered at all by wearing a baseball cap and allowing people to see that I have no hair, when there are some people who never go without a wig, even around their own families. And guess what? We're all coping. Being comfortable with yourself is coping. Not allowing baldness to interfere in your happiness is coping.

A few years back a friend told me that his mother had lost her hair several times, and eventually, it fell out and never came back. He said she took it very hard and refused to talk with anyone about it. She would not let anyone see her without a wig. She didn't even want to leave the house. I was determined that this was not going to happen to me. I was certain that I would never lose my hair forever, but if I did, I would not let it end my life. Well, I did lose my hair, it has not come back, and I can proudly say that I AM STILL ALIVE! When I found that my hair was not coming back, I read anything I could get my hands on that dealt with hair loss. My doctor gave me the address for the National Alopecia

Areata Foundation and I wrote to them and received some newsletters. I also read magazine articles. One of them was about a woman who had lost her hair due to alopecia, and as I read the article, everything about it screamed, "Victim!" I decided then and there that however emotionally crippling this disease was, I did not want to think of myself as a victim, hiding from the world, bitter and sad, scared to let anyone know me, much less see me.

My husband handles it quite well. He's never been anything but completely honest with me about everything, including my baldness. He knew of my condition when we met, and although I wasn't completely bald, he said it didn't bother him. God evidently knew what/who I needed when I met Doug. He has such a mature, unwavering love for me. But I must admit that I have a hard time trusting his word that my baldness doesn't turn him off. (Probably because it turns *me* off.) One of his favorite lines is, "I married you, not your hair." And he insists that he doesn't even "see it" anymore. He means that he looks at me, the person, not me, the hair.

Then why do I sometimes still feel insecure and ugly around him? The same reason that I sometimes feel insecure and ugly around others, including strangers. It all depends on how I'm feeling about myself. If I am feeling on top of things, confident, productive, active, it affects how I feel about me, which in turn affects how I feel about how others see me.

This is way too deep. I think it's far easier to believe the worst in oneself than to believe that we are worthy of acceptance. I find myself being overly critical in certain situations, like when we are being intimate. "Why won't he ever touch my head?" "Maybe he doesn't want to make me feel uncomfortable." "Maybe it turns him off." "Maybe he doesn't know he's not touching my head." "Why is he touching my head?" "To show me it doesn't make him uncomfortable?" "Maybe he doesn't know he's touching my head." "How could he NOT know he's touching my head? I know he's touching my head!" "Does he think I notice he's touching my head?" There. I've psychoanalyzed myself right out of the mood. "What, Honey? No, I just suddenly got a headache."

There were times when I was tempted to change the title of this book to "I Want to Make Love With My Hair. ...On." This is the time that I find not having hair the most distracting. Going to bed bald is ok, but one needs to create a picture of sexiness and confidence when initiating love making. In all honesty, I cannot picture myself bald while I'm "creating the picture," or else I lose all of my "creativity." And it's almost as difficult to do with a wig on, when *it* stays on the pillow *when you don't*. Or when in the throes of passion, your wig develops a mind of its own and begins to wander around on your head until you can't see, and covers your face, making you look like something out of "The Exorcist." Of course, there's always the alternative: you could hold your wig on with one hand, occasionally alternating when your hand falls asleep. Real sexy. And God forbid you should fall asleep with this wig on. You might dream you're being eaten head first by a big hairy monster, then wake up to the inside of your wig.

(Few people ever recover from this.) So you see- being intimate when you're bald is like being stuck between a rock and a hairy place. It either hurts, or it tickles, and I don't know whether to cry or laugh.

I sometimes feel like a pregnant woman, deep in hard labor, not knowing what she wants exactly, just wanting the pain to be over. A desperate woman shouting, *"Do* something! *Anything.* Don't do *that!"* "Rub my back!" "Don't touch me!" The poor man just can't please me. And yet there's nothing he can do. We both know that. Maybe tolerating my moods is one part of my ordeal he can take on now and then. It's pretty shameful of me to let him try, and sometimes I feel like a despicable human being, but I'm not. I'm just a human being. I have no control over what I feel or over my baldness. I DO, however, have control over how I *react* to what I feel. And that is where the challenge lies.

Being bald has definitely added new challenges to my life. Like what do I cover up when my hair blows off in the wind: my face or my head? And how do I ask someone to catch that hair ball rolling across the parking lot? How do I answer when children ask how my hair fell out? I really want to make it a profound, life-altering answer like, "This is what happens when you step on ants just for fun." Or, "This is what happens when you pick your nose." Or, "This is what you get for snooping in your mom's purse." But I just smile and tell them, "I don't know. It just fell out little by little when I brushed my hair. It's just this weird little disease that very few people get." And, "No, you can't catch it. (And if I **could** give it to someone, it would be that little snot who lived across the road from me when I was growing up. If ANYONE deserved to have this happen to them, it's her!) Ok. I'm over it. Which brings up a very good question, ALWAYS asked, NEVER answered. "Why ME?" Why not? I didn't say "why me?" when I found that twenty dollars... I don't know. And it doesn't matter. What matters is what I make of my situation. That is the deciding factor in whether it is a curse or a blessing. Making it a blessing is much more work than letting it be a curse. Why is depression, despair, and hopelessness so effortless? It is a constant struggle to maintain my belief that this is a blessing. (It's kind of like losing weight; it's a constant struggle to maintain the belief that I want to lose weight, which I don't- I just want to be a little thinner!) I can choose to either use it to help others and myself, or, at least, to not let it decide for me what I can and cannot do in my life. If I were to let it be a curse, I would just be lying down on the tracks and letting the train come. I would never be happy. Which brings me back to the challenges. It is truly a challenge, probably the greatest, to not be overcome with self-pity. Yes, there are disadvantages to having alopecia.

1. I can't use "washing my hair" as an excuse not to go out. Everyone knows I can leave my wet hair at home, and take my dry hair, or not wear hair at all.
2. I sneeze often, (no nose hairs to keep out the dust), but you know what they say about sneezing. (Next best thing to the "Big O." It's my favorite involuntary reflex!)

3. And because of no nose hairs, I also don't know when my nose is about to drip. HOW embarrassing.
4. I also bump my head more often. I don't know what the cause of this is.

    Maybe it has nothing to do with my being bald. Maybe I'm just clumsy. But ya know, I've heard a cat's whiskers are "feelers" of sorts. They know if a hole is too small to get through if their whiskers touch. So maybe my hairs were feelers! (But it will never serve the same purpose as a cat's whiskers. No matter how big I could "rat" my hair, it would never be as big as my butt. I'd get stuck every time.)
5. My expression can virtually disappear if I inadvertently rub off my eyebrows.
6. It's just damn inconvenient. Wigs can be itchy, and look stiff and too styled. Hats don't always stay on, and as a rule, don't cover baldness completely. Bandanas are just plain ugly. And what am I supposed to do when I go swimming at a public pool? I could wear one of those rubber swim caps with big daisies all over it…. or NOT…..
7. Without eyelashes, I am always getting dust and "stuff' in my eyes. (Not having eyelashes can also cause photosensitivity in some people, and more eye infections.)
8. Wind is enemy #1. (And a constant in the Midwest. They say if the wind ever stopped blowing, we'd all fall down.) If the wind *doesn't*

pluck the hair right off my head, roll it across the parking lot at the busiest mall in town and into the busiest street in town, bouncing it off several windshields of passing cars, causing severe psychological trauma and heart attacks and accidents, it simply makes me look like I've just been in a dog fight. With several big dogs. Licked without spit.
9. Did I mention the extraterrestrial qualities of my appearance?
10. And, of course, the most prevalent of all the disadvantages: I'm always cold during cooler months. (The other two months of South Dakota weather are stiflingly hot.)

See, there's a reason why U.T.S. is last on the list of cures- she can do lots of easy things to hide her unsightly malady: paint her toenails, wear shoes, walk faster... Alopecia is definitely worthy of a *little* more priority.

That's not to say that alopecia doesn't have it's advantages. I can think of a few

(grudgingly).

1. I save money because I don't have to buy hair-care products.
2. I can be ready to go out in the amount of time it takes some people to clean their ears.
3. I will never go gray. (Unless I want to...but who in their right mind would want to?)
4. If I don't like the hairstyle I just got, I just call

them up and order a different one. I don't have to wait for it to grow out.
5. It's not MY hair you just found in your food.
6. It's easier to pretend to be surprised about something if I just put my eyebrows on a little bit higher.
7. If I can't find my dogs or my cat, I have an instant pet with my wig if I'm feeling lonely and need to rub some fur. Just like my pets: always there, unconditional love, and a little static.
8. Instant Halloween costume! Wins the prize every time, no matter what I go as, because they think I'd go to any lengths to complete the look! And BTW, Winning ideas: Get pumped up, put in one loop earring, and go as Mr. (or Mrs.) Clean! Paint your head with glow-in-the-dark paint, paint your neck gray, instant light bulb! Put on your gray sweats, paint your head copper, you're a bullet!
9. No shaving! (except for those 5 hairs under my left armpit that sprout every now and then. And even though I feel it's a sin to shave ANY hair that may be the result of a prayer, I don't think these hairs will ever get long enough to comb over the top of my head.)
10. As soon as I come up with advantage #10, I'll get a hold of David Letterman.

I wasn't always this flip about being bald. I remember the first time I wore a wig in public. It looked like a German helmet. My husband took me out to eat after church that Sunday. It was a restaurant where I used to work. I felt I was safe there. Everyone there "knew." It was crowded. I was nervous. Doug assured me I looked fine. We greeted the hostess. So far, so good. I was feeling a little better. Then, from out of the kitchen, came John, a very uncool version of Tom Hanks. "Hey, Chris, NICE WIG!" and then he laughed. I died inside, and my outsides were quickly following suit. In an instant my face was hot, my eyes filled with tears, and I was frozen, mortified. I was certain every eye in the place was on me. There were lots of eyes that day. I wanted to turn right around and leave. Doug convinced me to stay, no one was even looking at me. I tried to believe him. All during lunch, I felt people staring at me. They weren't, of course. They had their own agendas. My hair was of no concern to them. But I still cried all during the meal. I couldn't eat a bite. One step forward, two steps back. How was I ever going to get through this? Fortunately, I never experienced anything like this again. No more German helmets for me.

I went through several wigs before I found one that I was completely happy with. When I attended my twenty-year class reunion, no one was any the wiser. Several people there made the comment that I looked as good as, or even better than, when I graduated! I was thrilled! Not so much about looking great after twenty years, (that was, however, my goal!), but because they noticed ME, not my hair, or lack of it.

I think I'm a fairly well-adjusted person now. I have my moments of feeling ugly and insecure. But I feel I have evolved from a scared, angry, bitter, sad, little lump into a beautiful (ok: relatively normal) creature. Reading back through the journals that I have kept since shortly before marrying Doug, I can recall vividly how I felt, not just about losing my hair or being bald, but all the "stuff" I was going through and how it may have affected me, and perhaps my immune system.

**11-3-86:**

Doug and I are getting along great. I love him so much I am thrilled just to hold him, touch him, kiss him. He makes me so happy. We had a good weekend- talked a lot, had fun. It's a miracle, finding him. My hair is falling out and I worry that one day he will be looking a different direction and not at me. He says he'll always love me. I know that. But how can I be sexy and alluring when all he can see is my bald head? What am I gonna do?! Some is coming back, but it's falling out fast. I don't want to go through all that again — God help me. I get so depressed about it and that doesn't help — it makes it worse. (Vicious circle.) Best go. Lots of work to do. (What's new?) Time to change.

**11-18-86:**

Had an awful two weeks. It's harvest, ya know. Don't see Doug much, see the kids too much. I'm still learning how to be a mom. Whew! It's work- I think I know why my hair falls out. When I get nervous, I fiddle with my hair & scratch my head & it comes out in handfuls! Major breakthrough, huh? So I cut off my fingernails & I'm buying Denorex & a soft bristle hair brush. Maybe, along with relaxing, this will work. We'll see! Best go!

**1-6-87:**

Me Again-..........Not much hair left to lose - I look sick. I don't know how Doug still finds me attractive. Even my eyelashes are falling out. I'm getting more depressed & crabby every day. And fat. Don't forget fat. I'll never be normal. I'll never be happy. I'll never be. Although suicide is scary, it looks more & more tempting every day. I have to get help. I went to Dr. Burrish yesterday, he did a biopsy on my head- 3 stitches-didn't hurt, (til I got home) just grossed me out. It sounded like he cut down to the bone. I'm so tired. Tired of feeling guilty, tired of being crabby, tired of thinking of me— I thought, Jesus, you never gave us more than we can handle?....

**2-2-87:**

Hello-.............Another day, another hand full of hair gone. I'm bald. A few hairs on top of my head. That's it. I look silly. I feel silly. But we have our laughs over it. And there are times I just can't handle it. I dream about hair every night. Why can't someone make a decent wig?! Maybe I should invent one. Get rich on my misfortune See ya.

**3-22-87:**

Hi- Haven't seen you for awhile............. Busy...........Maybe I don't turn him on any more.

.........Fat & Bald. Can't blame him ........I was crabby all day. Pissed off and depressed..

**7-3-87:**

Hello There! ......... 4th of July tomorrow! Whew! This year is flying! My hair is almost come in fully. A little left on the sides & behind the ears. Work is o.k..... Helped Doug yesterday and today........

**7-13-87:**

Hi. Guess I was little upset the other day. That's what you're here for. So maybe if I can let loose & get it all out, my hair won't fall out again, (fat chance.)

**10-87:**

Hi!....It's been awhile, eh? ........My hair is back. I look totally normal. Thank the <u>Dear Lord.</u>

**1-9-88:**

Hi!.................Been busy. Starting dieting—lost 6 lbs. so far............what I eat is healthy. I notice my pants are looser. I just pray I'm not being too hard on myself that I start losing my hair again. I'm taking vitamins—hope they work. I got so afraid today, I almost started crying. But I ate a big lettuce salad with a boiled egg. I'll be alright ........

**12-22-88:**

Hi- I'm depressed. I have two bald spots. I talked to John D. - his mom started out this way— losing hair every now & then. Then four years ago she lost it & it never came back. Now I'm beginning to think it could happen to me. Oh, God! What is causing this? I wish Doug was here. I'm at work & I really need him now. I'm so scared. Why me? Maybe it will always come back. Maybe it won't get any worse. Maybe I'll win 14.6 million in the Iowa Lottery! shit. Bye

**2-4-89:**

Hi Diary .......Remember me? The balding woman with saddlebags & baby blues? I hope it's soon—the Dr. said getting p.g. might help keep my hair in. It's going fast now. I'm sometimes worried & upset & obsessed & other times just thankful I have any hair yet Maybe my diet is the cause of my hair loss. I don't know. I'm tired of thinking about it.

**2-27-90:**

Hi, Bad-Weather Friend, ...Lots of Emotions Today! Things that are bothering me:
1) My hair is falling out again!

**8-2-93:**

Hello- Long time, eh? Well, I'm back to the land of the living. And I feel pretty good. As you know, I was in charter hospital. Suicidal, ya know. (Of course, you know!) It was getting pretty bad. But no one knew. Only you Life doesn't seem as pointless as before. But that doesn't mean I don't still see the dark side of things. My hair is gone. I'm handling that ok, (I think) "Oh, Well" I hope it comes back!

**8-10-93:**

Hi, Still me- still bald- still neurotic. Oh, well

I haven't made mention of my lack of hair in my diary since then. I don't write in it as much as I once did. However, journaling still helps me immensely. I write whenever something is bothering me, or when something has had a profound effect on me. It's good therapy and "it" seems to know when "it" is needed. No judgments, no opinions, no lectures. There are many secrets within those pages, thus, my family has strict instructions to burn it unread should anything happen to me. Sometimes it's not as therapeutic writing it as it is reading it later. It's easier to understand things once you're removed from it.

I suppose the only thing journal-worthy on the subject of my hair loss would be my dreams of having hair. Waking up from one of these dreams is like losing my hair all over again, but much faster. I find I have these dreams after daydreaming about my hair coming back, or after my hopes are lifted upon hearing about a new treatment. I remember so many dreams of having hair, long and curly, short and bouncy, all different colors, my dreams are not fussy, any hair will do. In my dreams, I'm aware that I have alopecia, but now I have hair, and I'm so thankful! I love it! I brush it, style it, (NEVER cut it), fling it over my shoulder, let it hang in my face, (my mother would have a fit and fall in it!), throw it around, feel it cool and soft on my neck and back, run my fingers through it, and adore it in the mirror, all the while smiling. I'm so happy! Then I wake up.

It was just a dream. Damn! Why do I have to dream about it! This is not helping me accept my hair loss! I'd cry, be angry all over again, be moody all day, mourn my hair loss. Again. But not now.

Before I tell you why it's different now, let me tell you of a conversation I had with my husband. One time, a year ago or so, I told Doug that I'm not sure how I'd feel if my hair came back. Of course, I'd be excited and grateful. But would there be so much fear and anxiety overshadowing my excitement that I'd literally make it fall out again? Wouldn't it be harder to get it back just to lose it again, if that is what is to be? How could I handle this again? I don't know if I *could* handle losing my hair again. Maybe I don't want it back if it's only going to be temporary. It would be easier to stay bald than to relive all that pain over and over again. Doug just sat and listened. When I was done carrying on needlessly over this hypothetical situation, Doug said, "I think it would be best to just think of your hair, however temporary, as a gift. A time that you wouldn't have to wear a wig. A time to just have your hair. Nothing else. Whatever happens, happens. You'll deal with it." He was so right. (He's such a wise man! I think in his past life he was a ..... what do you call them? ... a wise man. Maybe one of *the* wise men.)

And it wasn't until perhaps two months ago that I realized the same applied to my dreams. Maybe dreaming about hair was my little gift to myself. Maybe, however short or unreal this time with hair was, I needed to think of it as a way to have hair - any kind of hair I wanted - to feel the same things, to see the same things, to have the same things that everyone with hair has. Now I recall how I felt in my dreams, how my hair felt, how fun it was to have hair. And when I have dreams about hair, and I wake up, I may, for a moment, be a little saddened that it was only a dream, but then I can say I had hair, if only in my dreams, and it was fun while it lasted.

**5-18-97**

Hi! ...You wouldn't believe what I dreamed about last night! Yup! Hair! Yesterday I was writing in the chemo chapter of my book, mentioning how I sometimes plan for my future hair. I must've been fantasizing a bit too much, because I had a dream that I had hair. In my dream, I went into the bathroom, brushed my short, dark, silky, bouncy hair, and walked into the dining room to surprise everyone with my "new" hair. They all thought it was a wig, saying it was beautiful, it looked so real, it felt so real, etc. I told them it *was* real! One of them asked, "When did it begin to grow in?" I thought about it: I didn't have it a couple days ago, I didn't have it yesterday, Wait a minute.

Hair like this doesn't grow overnight. THIS IS A DREAM!!!! Damn!! And I started to cry. In my dream. I knew I was dreaming, I knew I would be bald when I woke up. Janelle O., in my dream, said, "Remember, Chris, this is a gift. Right now you have hair."

I bucked up and said, "That's right," and finished my dream enjoying my hair. When I woke up, I looked over at Doug, and I just laughed. That was so bizarre

I can't even believe it. Reality invades my fantasy. Oh, well, at least I had hair.

## "Lexie"

*When I was seven years old, in second grade, I lost three patches of hair. One the size of a penny, another, a nickel, and the third, a quarter. When my parents discovered the spots, we went to the doctor for a check. The doctor told us it was normal for children my age to lose hair and that it should grow back. He was right and it all came back Two years lapsed without any of my hair falling out.*

*Unfortunately, the time came again that I had patches of hair missing. But these patches did not fill in. They slowly grew and eventually my head was bald. I also lost my eyebrows, bottom eyelashes, and arm and leg hair. My parents rushed me to the doctor, only to be told that there was no cure, just treatments. We tried creams, but there was no way to tell if they were working, or if my hair was growing in naturally. All we had was a name for this condition: Alopecia Areata. Most of my hair returned, minus a few hidden spots. Although my original appearance returned, I had changed. Fourth graders can be cruel. At a stage [in life] where girls want to wear makeup and different hairstyles, appearance makes a world of difference. From that point on, I have never been secure with my appearance.*

*My hair remained during the following year, but sixth grade brought more hard times. The small patches overtook my scalp once again. This time was more difficult. Sixth grade boys and girls begin to notice each other and take an interest in each other. My regular doctor recommended I see a psychiatrist* because my alopecia might be stress related. If anything, the alopecia brought the stress into my life. After a few months, I was labeled "normal" without any stress. I continued with the creams, but still had no idea if they were making a difference. There was no way to tell if the treatments helped or if my hair growth was natural. Crude things were said to me. The people I went to school with never commented, but those who knew nothing of my condition were not pleasant. The unusually long stares and hushed comments were enough to do damage. For some reason, people seem to think that when you are bald you can't see them staring or hear their comments. Once again, in the spring, my hair returned. It wasn't a full head of hair, but it covered my white scalp.

Fall of my seventh grade year brought more difficulties. A pattern had started to develop. I would lose my hair in the fall and it would start to grow back in the spring. Although it had a cycle, it wasn't any easier. Losing hair is never easy. You can never be prepared enough. This was the year that I began to wear wigs. My parents and I decided to give those a try along with the combination of medicines. It was awkward at first, but eventually wearing a wig made being in public easier. Fewer people noticed so I received less stares. I did overhear comments made by my classmates concerning a few practical jokes, but I chose to ignore them. Luckily, none of them followed through.

That year I had one really embarrassing moment. During a basketball game, I was bumped in the head, which caused my wig to fall off. The referee stopped the game, which made the situation worse because everyone had the chance to stare. All I wanted to do was go home and hide. Although I didn't believe it at the time, I'm glad I stayed in the game. Actually, I was forced to play because my team wouldn't have had enough players if I had left. Staying taught me that I couldn't let my wig or my alopecia run my life. I was still a regular kid.

My hair never grew back in eighth grade. I got a new wig and used that as my solution. It was an easier year. I had no reason to get my hopes up that my hair would return. I also didn't have to worry about it falling out again. That spring my family went to Florida for a traditional Disney trip. It was extremely hot and my wig was unbelievably uncomfortable. One day I decided to go without it. Nothing could have prepared me for the looks I received that day. After all, I definitely didn't look like the average kid. I was even asked if I was there through the "Make a Wish Foundation."

When I look back on it, that day brought a huge revelation in my life. I realized that my life could be a lot worse. I could've been sick, maybe from cancer and been receiving chemotherapy. Instead, I was just bald. Sometimes it's important to look at where you are and where you could be.

Our eighth grade graduation party was held at a country club and the festivities included swimming. When I took my wig off, I just got a few quick glances. In general, my classmates knew about my situation and didn't comment. They just wanted to know what I looked like without a wig. I wasn't treated any differently.

The switch from junior high to high school wasn't what I expected. People I didn't know knew about my condition. I wasn't ready for the questions. Mostly they would ask if I wore a wig or if I had a weave, but most people didn't bother to ask why. They all assumed there was some story, but it couldn't possibly be that interesting. I never let the condition stop me from participating in any activities. I always told myself that alopecia wouldn't ruin or run my life. I participated in numerous activities and never had a problem with my alopecia interfering.

I ordered wigs in different colors and styles. Some curly, some straight, short, long, light or dark brown. They wore out quickly, but I was usually ready for a change every few months. The summer after my junior year I spent in Wisconsin. While I was there I stopped wearing my wig. After three bad years, my hair was healthy and covered my scalp fairly well. I returned home with a new confidence. I was more sure of myself. I even had my senior pictures taken without a wig, which to me meant that I wouldn't wear a wig at school. Everyone I went to school with already knew about my condition. I never wore wigs to hide it or pretend that I didn't have alopecia. I wore them so that people I didn't know wouldn't stare or make comments. Strangers were always worse about it. When you go to school with the same kids for 10 years, they are bound to know even if you don't tell them.

My senior year went well. My hair pretty much stayed intact. I decided to try a new treatment that spring to fill the areas that were still empty. Unfortunately, it was a very painful process. I never had a problem getting shots, but cortisone injections were not what I expected. I received 200 to 300 shots on my scalp once a month. It hurt and itched and some spots even bled. Once again the treatment didn't produce any results. But I was prepared for it not to work. I had learned not to get my hopes up, in any case, no matter what the doctors said.

During my senior year, there was a new fad where teenagers shaved the hair at the base of their head. I looked like I had done this since I was basically missing the hair underneath. My confidence level was still rather high. I didn't have many choices for hair styles because pulling my hair back or up revealed my bare scalp. But I felt lucky to have the amount of hair I had. I was a lifeguard the following summer, which also raised my confidence. It was another thing I had always wanted to do and I was very determined not to let my alopecia stand in my way. Very few people noticed it or had the nerve to say anything about it. Exposure to the sun was also supposed to be good for my scalp.

My hair remained healthy and I started college at USD. I was definitely nervous about that. It's hard enough to be comfortable starting college, but to go with a physical difference made it worse. I was especially worried about what my roommate would think. Fortunately, she was spectacular about it and even said she hadn't really noticed. My hair did thin out that year, but not too drastically. My friends were very supportive and helped me through a few bad hair days. During that year, I stopped receiving treatments. They didn't seem to be making a difference and the pain definitely wasn't enjoyable. The year flew by without any major traumatic experiences.

That summer, I had the opportunity to attend the National Alopecia Areata Foundation Conference. I met so many people with the same problems. I also realized that I handled the situation differently than quite a few people. So many of them let it decide what they were allowed to do. Many of them hid like they had a disease that might be contagious and make them different from the rest of the world. Other people were very outspoken. Almost obnoxious about it, making sure everyone they met knew about it. I guess their attitudes were as diverse as the levels of alopecia.

My sophomore year in college wasn't quite as smooth. During November, my hair took a turn for the worse. It slowly, but consistently fell out. My mid-February, it was practically gone. I had one strip on the top and one across the back. They basically formed and upside down "T." At this point, I really turned to my sorority sisters for support. I decided to shave it off completely. One of my sisters actually shaved it for me. Everyone was very encouraging. In fact, most of them said it looked better shaved that when it had been so thin. It was pretty easy to adjust. It took me no time to get ready in the morning. I got plenty of compliments. Apparently when you don't have any hair, people direct their attention elsewhere.

I shaved it weekly, from February through April. Then miraculously, my hair started to grow thicker. I decided to stop shaving it because I wanted to have hair for my sister's wedding. I had straight hair before, but this time it was curly. It was darker than ever, but it did start to lighten up. I didn't really care about the color or style as long as I had hair. It slowly grew in and started to cover my scalp.

In September, a few areas slowly started falling out again. For the most part it is still growing healthily. I started treatment again with pills and creams. That brings us up to date. Everyday I wonder if it will fall out again or if by chance all of it will grow back. I haven't lost all hope, but I have accepted the fact that I probably won't ever have a full head of hair. Alopecia is just so unpredictable. Every case is so different. I'm just lucky to have some hair. I'm also lucky to have the opportunity to try different treatments. Maybe one of these days something will work.

Having alopecia has definitely had a severe impact on my life. I know that it has made me a better person. I know that I am less judgmental of people's looks. I never stare if someone has an abnormality. After all, I know exactly how that feels.

*The stares are incredibly embarrassing and the comments hurt more than anyone could imagine. Everyone wants to fit in and it's harder when you look different.*

When I was younger, I had a very difficult time dealing with my alopecia. More than once, I shut myself out from people. I didn't want to talk about it, even with my family. Sometimes you just want to hide and pretend that this problem will go away. But it doesn't work. I tried to hard not to let it bother me. But in a world where so much emphasis is placed on appearance, it's practically impossible to ignore how you look, especially when other people constantly remind you.

I do think that having alopecia made me grow up faster. Yes, I am bitter about that. When other kids were worried about sports and school, I had so much more to worry about. I dealt with doctor after doctor and treatment after treatment. I also had to learn not to get my hopes up, because every time I did, they would be crushed. I never took false hope from the doctors either, and they never tried to give me any. I was constantly reminded that alopecia is very unpredictable. There are no guarantees with the medications that I took. What worked for one patient probably wouldn't work for me. My case was so extreme.

Never once did I take my hair for granted. We celebrated the slightest changes. For example, my mom threw a party for me at school the first time my hair started to grow back. We had strawberry shortcake with my entire class. We even celebrated when my eyebrows and bottom eyelashes grew back. One definite advantage was that we never had to celebrate the hair on my legs growing back. Not having to shave is definitely a plus. But that is just me thinking on the positive side. Always looking for the best in every situation.

As for my support system, I never would have survived without my family. My parents made sure that I knew how much they loved me, no matter what I looked like. They took me to doctor after doctor, including specialists at the Mayo Clinic, looking for an answer. I got to try every treatment. They kept me on track with my medications and tried to keep up my spirits. They were there to laugh with me, and cry. I shed so many tears. They dealt with all my moods, too. I was about as unpredictable as my alopecia. My siblings were wonderful, also. I got quite a bit of attention from a lot of people because I looked different. But they handled it pretty well. They were never embarrassed to be seen with someone who got quite a few stares. They also told me that they didn't care what I looked like. My extended family was always concerned. When I raised money for the National Alopecia Areata Foundation, they were very generous with hopes that the research would finally help me. They especially liked all the new hairdos each time they saw me. And they always wanted updates on my condition. The support of my family really got me through some tough times.

As for my friends, things weren't always so cheery. I do have a few friends that have stood by me from day one and are still here when I need them. Each time my hair fell out, I had friends who practically ran away. As I said before, I did shut myself out from people at times, which made friendships difficult. But more than once, I overheard comments from some of my so-called friends. I guess I've accepted that fact that kids are like that. As I've gotten older, I've heard fewer comments. I know I have the support of everyone that is around me now. Maybe it's just the change of going to college and being around more mature people. I have had a few rude things said to me, but for the most part I believe that people are a little more mature and informed.

One thing that really bothered me and still does today is when people call alopecia a disease. I've never heard anyone with alopecia call it a disease before. Probably because it sounds like we are sick and possibly contagious. Alopecia is a condition. It affects the immune system and nothing else and it definitely isn't contagious. To me, disease is a nasty sounding word. Another thing that still bothers me, is how people treat me differently because they think I am ill. Most people just assume that, rather than finding out the real story. I also really hate the pity I receive. Although no one has ever said the actual words, "I pity you," it was pretty easy to see it in their faces. I never asked for pity or sympathy. They only made the situation worse.

The easiest way for me to deal with this situation is to tell people about it. I really appreciate the people who have the courage and courtesy to ask me about it, rather than make assumptions. Alopecia is common, but there are very few people in this area that have it. The more people know about it, the easier it is for me to deal with it.

My advice for anyone who has alopecia is to look for the positives. Just remember: "Bald is beautiful. God only made so many perfect heads, the others He covered with hair." I guess I should be thankful; I've been told quite a few times that my head is perfect to be bald. When you don't have hair, your other features get more attention.

*Lexie"*

## On Men and Alopecia

It was my goal to include a variety of personal accounts

from all types of people experiencing hair loss, including, but not limited to, those with alopecia. However, I found that during my efforts to include men in this cross section of the population, I encountered more of an unwillingness to "pour out their hearts" on paper. While some men would not object to answering my questions, or sending me a simple statement of their experience, I discovered that men, in general, would not allow themselves to seem emotional about their experience with alopecia.

I know or know of several men who have alopecia and have profound or total hair loss. When I asked these men if they would be interested in sharing their story with others, none of them outwardly objected. But then again, after waiting and waiting, I also did not discover many letters from them in my mailbox. Therefore, I can only share with you what I do have, and speculate on the rest.

## "Bob"

*My name is Bob. I am married and self-employed. I am 33 years old. I first noticed my hair falling out about a year ago, when chunks of my beard started to fall out and I had dry, red, flakey skin where the hair was falling out. I had real(ly) long hair. It was down to my waist, very strong, and healthy, but every time I combed my hair, the brush was full of hair.*

*After about five months of this, my hair was so thin, I just shaved it all off. When it was coming back, it was salt & pepper color. I let it grow for about a month and the dark hair was still falling out, so I shaved it again with the hope of it all coming back and staying.*

*Now my mustache is falling out and my eyebrows are getting thinner. Nothing has changed in my life, and no change in my living habits or diet. Thank you for listening to my story.*

"Bob" seems to be coping quite well with his baldness. He doesn't hide his baldness, and he doesn't seem embarrassed to talk about it. It's not a big "issue" in his life.

Hair loss, however, can be an issue to those who *seem* to be coping. There is a man who lives not far from me who began to lose his hair about three years ago. He is 60-ish, tall, good-looking, outgoing, successful, but when he began to lose his hair, he did everything he could to keep it. He was self-conscious about his hair loss, and wore a hat whenever possible. When it was apparent that he was fighting a losing battle, he quit the treatments and today his hair continues to thin. And although he talked openly with me *when I asked him about it,* he was reluctant to write about it. And the same goes with the other four or five men I met who had alopecia totalis or universalis. We all cope in different ways. As with "Bob," some men shaved their heads and preferred to not deal with hair at all, where others had full cranial hair pieces. All the men with alopecia that I met were active in society, working at their jobs, active in their relationships, their churches, their social lives, and were otherwise healthy and happy. And I'd say they're all dealing with hair loss the right way: coping in a way that each of them is comfortable with, and getting on with their lives.

Chapter Eight

# The Naked Truth
Options for hair-challenged people.

Hard as I try, I can't help feeling somewhat naked without something- hair, hat, scarf, whatever- on my head when greeting someone other than my husband and children. I've come to believe that hair was created for other practical purposes besides the obvious. I now believe it was intended also to break up the great expanses of skin. If having a naked head isn't enough, try removing every stitch of clothing *along* with having no hair at all. Talk about exposure!! Now *that's* naked! If it weren't for the jewelry that I never remove, I'd look like I was literally *dipped* in skin. A great big, pink, skin-coated cookie. An oversized, flesh-colored, human "Turtle" candy. (You get the picture.)

I don't believe that I have a distorted self-image. I have a mirror. I know what I look like. I know I'm not ugly. I just like what hair does for human beings, myself included. Too much hair could be as disconcerting and distracting, but that's a different show.

If you're anything like me, and you'd like your face to end above your forehead and not behind it, then you probably want to know what your choices are for head coverings and face enders. I'll start with hair since that is what we lack and yearn for most.

## WIGS..........

Wigs come in as many styles and prices as humans do. Lucky for you, you can pick just what you want! Your physician or dermatologist can point you in the direction of a salon in your area that deals with medically related hair loss if you have alopecia or hair loss from chemo. And many barbers and salons also fit men with hair pieces in the case of male pattern baldness.

Probably the least expensive wigs are those that are mail order, averaging between 30 and 80 dollars. That does not mean, however, that they are all "cheap." I've found some very satisfactory wigs in mail order catalogs, such a Paula Young, Revlon, Dolly Parton, Beauty Trends, Adolfo, to name a few. One Alopecian mentioned, though, that she felt that these wigs "were not made for bald people." While I tend to agree that these wigs are generally generic in style and make and some can look "wiggy" or have a helmet or "big hair" appearance, they more than deliver a sense of normalcy and security to one who has no hair and not a lot of money. And in the case of chemo hair loss, most often temporary and relatively short term, mail order wigs are very practical.

These mail order wigs are very affordable and easy to care for, and I've been extremely impressed with the quality of customer service and speedy delivery they offer. Once you get your mail order wig, if it seems to have too much hair, or doesn't look as natural as you'd like, you can return it, or if you choose to keep it, you can even take it to your local hair salon and have a professional hair dresser thin it out and style it while you wear it.

Synthetic (man-made) hair is basically plastic so naturally you cannot use a hair dryer, curling iron, hot rollers or anything that can generate heat. These wigs will melt as fast as a bread wrapper against a toaster. Even leaning over a hot stove or open oven door can melt them. So be sure your hair dresser understands exactly what she's dealing with. And since this hair does not grow back if the stylist goofs, most stylists will hesitate to offer any kind of guarantees or promises. And of course, the wig is not returnable once you alter it, so be sure of what you want.

The care of these wigs is minimal- you can wash it in the bathroom sink with special wig shampoo, also available through these mail order catalogues, which is specifically made for synthetic hair. Synthetic hair, just like real hair or anything you wear on your head on a regular basis, is going to collect dirt and absorb body oils. You will also need to use on these synthetic wigs only hair spray specially made for synthetic hair.

Regular hair sprays contain ingredients that damage, and are extremely difficult to wash out of, synthetic hair. You can usually find small ads in the back of your favorite magazines telling you where to get a copy of these mail order wigs. (I'm not absolutely sure if "Field & Stream" can accommodate you in this area.)

Unfortunately, these mail order catalogues do not cater to men. Since men generally wear their hair shorter than women, it's more difficult to naturalize a hairpiece, especially when it needs to be made to blend in with existing hair. Men would benefit more from going to a hair replacement center and being fitted with a custom hair piece, sized and styled to their exact needs. And for men who suffer profound hair loss, whether it be male-pattern baldness, alopecia, or whatever, it is possible to find very realistic hair replacements, or prostheses. (read on.)

There are disadvantages to using mail order catalogues to purchase wigs or hair pieces. First of all, hair color is hard to match just by looking at a picture of a few strands of hair. No representative is ever going to be able to describe exactly what color you are asking about, or be able to match hair color to your own over the telephone. They can be very helpful and patient, but phone conversations will never replace the human factor. It is also very apparent that these are fashion wigs, not catering to children or young adults. The sizes and styles prohibit use by youth. Some of them come in S-M-L, but most are "Average Head Size." These wigs are made of elastic bands with hair sewn onto them called "wefting", and have adjustable bands in the back. The longer styles can become matted and tangled, and after awhile become harder to manage, style, and naturalize, getting a "hard" look. I also know from personal experience that this type of wig can be itchy, ill-fitting, and hard to secure on one's head. But, again, they are well worth the minimal investment, especially if you like to change your hair style often, or even your hair color! You could have a lot of fun being the blonde, brunette, or redhead you've always wanted to be - all in the same week! I recall reading about one Alopecian who did just that. All her coworkers knew of her alopecia and loved the surprises she gave them by coming to work with a different look now and then. Why not take advantage of the opportunity to present a different you, a daring you, a wilder you! I'm not suggesting that you run right out and have "Born to be Wild!" tattooed on your.... BUT, you might be surprised at what a different look can do for your self-esteem. In the case of alopecia, where the length of time without hair can be uncertain, I would definitely recommend this type of inexpensive wig with which to begin. Many people who have alopecia regrow their hair spontaneously months or even years after it fell out. But for someone without hair, every day can be an eternity. Be sure of what you want before investing in the more expensive hairpieces. The cost of a good wig, or hair prosthesis, can range from a few hundred to a few thousand dollars. Much of that depends on whether the hair is human or synthetic, if the wig is custom fit mesh, fiberglass or vinyl with hard or soft vacuum fit, which brings us to a new level of hair-ness.

    Thanks to the NAAF, through their efforts to make the public more aware of alopecia and other medical related hair losses, research is not only being done on hair loss itself, but the alternatives to baldness. Many companies have sprouted throughout the country that cater to those who have profound hair loss and they have developed some truly amazing products. No, I'm not talking about the "Hair-in-a-Spray-Can" thing.

Several years ago, I heard of a woman named Peggy Knight who had a hand in revolutionizing the wig industry. She, along with a woman named Raine Davidson, helped to develop a wig, more aptly named prosthesis, that was actually molded to the exact fit of the individual for whom the wig was being made. It is made so precisely that it will not come off in the wind, or during sleep, or even when swimming. Just like Tupperware, it has a vacuum fit, and the only way it comes off is to break the vacuum. They are made with human hair, and the hair is implanted in the cap to give the look of hair growing from the scalp. These wigs can be cut, styled, and permed. Most everything that you could do to a real head of hair, you can do to these. (And as an added bonus, you can take them off when you are going to sort pigs, and put them back on when you're done! Do THAT with a real head of hair!) Of course, nothing is perfect and naturally they could come off if you were in football and took a hard hit, but considering all the challenges that go along with wigs, this was a Godsend. Vacuum wigs are custom made to fit the individual's head only. To make these vacuum wigs, a plaster mold is made of the head, and then the wig cap is made from that mold. These bases are tinted to replicate actual scalp color. Then hair is injected by hand into a flexible base that is then glued onto this cap. Talk about labor-intensive! But this is truly a labor of love - even though this type of hair replacement is expensive, it is the closest thing to a real head of hair some of us will ever have. And I, for one, am glad that there are dedicated workers who are willing to do this to make others' lives a little easier.

Over the years, the idea and the wig, or prosthesis, was perfected. They are now made thinner, more flexible, and more available. There are many companies that now make and sell their own version of this type of wig. You can find custom-made cranial prostheses in vacuum type, made with vinyl or fiberglass hard and soft bases, and also custom made mesh bases. You can even specify whether you want human hair, synthetic hair, or a combination of both. What more could you ask for? How about more money? I have not been able to justify this expense yet. I'm "just" a housewife, and my pay leaves much to be desired. I'm not even saying I'm not worth it. But if I worked outside the home, (outside, not meaning in the hog house, sorting pigs,) I would give this type of hair piece serious consideration. When I do go away from home, and I wear my wig, almost all I can think about is getting home and taking my hair off. It would be such a joy to wear something on my head that looked natural, felt comfortable and not so foreign, and was relatively worry-free. (See the P.S. below!)

Vacuum-fit prostheses, custom-fit wigs, and hairpieces are widely available for all types of people, young and old alike. Yes, they are expensive, but the fact that they are considered a "prosthesis" instantly qualifies them as necessary and you may be able to use your insurance to help pay for one. Some states require insurance carriers, including health maintenance organizations, to pay for portions of the expenses toward a hair prosthesis, or medical treatment. Contact your current health insurance representative and have them research it for you, and do not be too quick to take "no" for an answer. Most insurance companies expect you to accept this answer without rebuttal, and ultimately, they benefit from this tactic or "policy." It would definitely be worth your time and effort to pursue compensation. (See the next chapter for more information on this.)

Lastly, on the subject of vacuum and custom fit wigs, hairpieces, and prostheses, be certain to talk to a professional who deals with these types of hair replacements, and for that matter, talk with several professionals. (Shop around- this is a costly investment.) They can explain the care and benefits, as well as the drawbacks and expenses, of their product. Ask about guarantees, their credentials, references, and training in maintenance and styling of the hair replacement.

PS. When I wrote this book, and eventually finished it, I had not yet bought the vacuum wig that I have now. I felt it was important to add to this segment rather than delete parts of my previous information so you would know my true feelings before and after getting a vacuum wig. My husband gave it to me as a Christmas gift. How do I like it? Let me just say how very GLAD I am that Christ was born!! It was the best gift (besides forgiveness) that I've ever been given. "Way, Way Up There" kind of gift. Right up there with the dishwasher, electric blanket, coffee grinder, and The Big Chill movie. Is it comfortable? I often answer this question by telling people it's like wearing a comfortable pair of tennis shoes. If you think about it, you can feel it. But for the most part, you forget it's there. Eventually you stop grabbing your head when the wind comes up or you have to bend over. You can part your hair on either side. You can comb one side without holding the other. You can feel it cool and soft on the back of your neck. Even after I tell people it's a wig, they refuse to believe it. It's very realistic, easy to care for, and comfortable. I would highly recommend it. Again, check around for the best prices and references.

## HATS:

If you don't care to wear a wig, or can't afford one, you still have options. There is always the hat. Now don't go off and say right away, "I'm not a hat person. I can't wear hats." Poo. It's not the hat or you. It's how you present yourself. Anyone can wear hats. If you put one on and act like you don't care who sees you or what they think, you are a hat person.

Now that we have that cleared up, let's talk about where and what. Hats are sold just about everywhere that you can buy clothing. "Ball" caps, with a bill, are very popular and comfortable. These don't cover all of your head, but other than a wig or a full head of hair, almost nothing can hide the fact that you don't have any hair. Ball caps work great for working outdoors or when you're wearing jeans, something casual. But it's at those times when you care least about your hairlessness. The times you really care about are when you're going shopping, going visiting, holidays, appointments, going to work, and evenings out. There are hats for every occasion. Big and fancy, plain and simple, cotton, denim, velvet, velour, whatever you please. Hats with big flowers on the front are very popular right now. I guess I don't wear these as often, but I do have a white dressy straw hat with a daisy on the front. I wear it with a black and white shorts outfit and it *makes* the outfit. So you see, a hat can actually detract from your baldness. If it helps make a total statement with your outfit, people notice "the look," not so much the baldness. My favorite is a black velvet "tam." It's elasticized around the bottom and is slightly floppy and has a matching bow in front. My family calls it my "artist" hat. It's not really appropriate for summer wear, but it gets a workout the rest of the year. You just need to be the judge of what you're comfortable with, what hat is proper for what occasion, and go with it.

Some wig catalogues and retailers also deal in hats and turbans. I even found a catalogue that deals strictly with hats. It's called Paula's Hatbox, address, P.O. Box 935, South Easton, MA. They have just about every hat you could need.

Probably the only thing you need to keep in mind when you're wearing a hat is to make it fit the occasion or coordinate with your outfit. Hats can be worn for any event that hair can be worn. As a matter of fact, there was once a time when a woman wouldn't be caught dead without a proper hat. It was also the same era in which gloves were commonplace and necessary to a woman's wardrobe. Fortunately, hats have survived the times and as long as there are heads, there will also be hats. (I think it's safe to say that hats will be around a while.)

You'll probably decide right off what types of hats you will NOT wear. That's cool. Pick what you like, and you'll be comfortable wearing it. My main goal in wearing hats is it's easy, it's quick, it's relatively worry and fuss free, but mostly I wear hats when I'm around home working because I prefer comfort over looks most of the time, although I also don't want to shock people with my great white head. It's not even that important to me to conceal the fact that I'm bald. I don't care who knows. I don't care who sees, even though I don't care to stand out like a sore thumb, either. Now, if Clint Eastwood happened to be walking my way, I might duck into a doorway, put on my wig, lipstick, sexy evening gown, and very high heels. (I LOVE that man.) Incidentally, my husband looks a lot like him. Lucky me! Anyway, if you're like me, you *sometimes* like to be the life of the party and have fun, but for the most part, just like to fit in - be just another face. To do that, you must be comfortable with yourself. When we're not feeling confident and comfortable, we fidget, don't look people in the eye, don't go out of our way to be social, avoid people we know, yadda, yadda, yadda. I hate that feeling. It's not the wig or the hat that's responsible for these feelings. It's the way we see ourselves and it's not a fair assessment because that's not how others see us.

## AU NATUREL:

Someday I hope to have enough confidence to go au naturel'. The only way I can do this and feel that I am acceptable in the public's eye is if I make a complete statement with my clothing, jewelry, makeup, and accessories. I simply cannot picture a woman in a navy business suit, white silk blouse, matching shoes and panty hose, and conservative gold jewelry walking into a board meeting completely bald and NOT being conspicuous. However, if a woman wore more unconventional, flowing, or chic clothing, bright colors, fun jewelry, and accentuating makeup, the bold, naked head would go right along with it. Accessorize! After all, you don't have anything that everybody else doesn't have. *Everyone* is bald under their hair. Just like everyone is naked under their clothing. Remember that old stage fright trick, "Think of everyone naked and you won't be so scared." Same holds true for hair. Only difference is, you ARE naked (in a sense). BUT, *"nee-ner, nee-ner,"* there's no law against it! Could even be fun! Liberating! Sensual! And eventually, within your own circle of friends, in your own community, your bald head will cease to exist in everyone's eyes. It just needs to cease to exist in your own eyes first. BIG first.

One of my fellow Alopecians, who lives in a large city, said that after she lost all her hair, she became almost defiant and went everywhere bald. While bigger cities tend to be more accepting of radical looks, that doesn't mean that Beresford, SD, population: 1800, or your town or community, couldn't get used to it. Besides, it's not your responsibility to make everyone *else* comfortable. If you're comfortable going out without anything on your head, then that's all that matters. You deserve to feel just as comfortable as the rest of the general public feels with and about their head. Tip: *If you're* comfortable, *you're* coping. Don't let someone else's idea of "coping" determine what you should be doing. In several articles and talk shows featuring baldness, women -and men-declared that they were "free" from society's expectations of them. I got the feeling that they were implying that because I was not going everywhere bald, that I was denying my "uniqueness" and I wasn't coping. They were going to go out bald, they were determined and righteous and proud! Bravo! Good for them! I can be just as proud with a baseball cap. I must admit that I get tired of the never-ending unsolicited advice, sympathetic hugs, and curious stares. Sometimes I just want to blend in, not be noticed, not get moved to the head of the checkout because they think my time is running out right there at Target. (As if I would go shopping if I had mere minutes to live!) No! I'd go out to eat!! Anyway, just do what makes you feel good or comfortable.

There is a practical side to wearing hats, wigs, scarves, turbans, and the like. In the winter, over 60% of your body heat escapes from your head. Bet you didn't know your brain could generate that much energy, huh? Also, besides looking kinda neat, hair IS instrumental in protecting you from other elements such as the sun. Too much exposure to the hot sun, with or without hair, can cause heat stroke. Without hair, your risks are much higher. You also run a great risk of getting a nasty sunburn. I've tried, but my scalp doesn't want to tan very easily. So I've found that it's safer and more comfortable to wear a cap or something on my head when I'm going to be outdoors for any length of time. So, if you do decide to go au naturel', do it smart. Protect your tender head.

For those of you who have children with alopecia or any other type of profound hair loss, be especially careful with their tender, bare heads. Use sun blocks *and* protective headwear on them.

As well as *being* bald, covering one's bald head has many challenges.

Wigs, no matter how expensive or ingenious, can come off when you least expect it. Hats can be uncomfortable and ill-fitting, spinning around on top of your head like a propeller, but the only other choice you have besides going "topless" is turbans and scarves. Both leave much to be desired in terms of fashion, but can be the most comfortable things our weary heads can get. Granted, the turban, especially the terry-cloth type, give the "patient-undergoing-treatment" look, but for around home they're priceless. You can even buy little snippets of hair to attach to these turbans to give the appearance of bangs. (And by the way, where did that word come from, "bangs?" Do those little wisps of hair *bang* our foreheads? No. Are they *for* banging? Hardly. It's probably got Latin roots. Get it? Roots? I'm probably the only one who laughs at my jokes. Say it once. "Bangs." Must be German. "Bangs." Not a very pretty word. Say it a few times. "Bangsbangsbangsbangsbangsbangs...". Is it even a word? I say no. Come to think of it, I recall vaccinating our cattle for a disease called "Bangs." And if you only had one hair on your forehead, like Charlie Brown, would it be called a "Bang?") Moving right along....

As far as scarves go, there is always the bandana, quite unattractive on a naked head, but very functional. (Band-aids are quite functional, too, but that doesn't mean I want to show them off.) I have expanded my scarf wardrobe to include the longer, silky scarves in various weights. I buy them at least 10 inches wide and 4 feet long, pretty standard size. I wrap them from the back of my head to the front, crossing the ends above my forehead, wrap them to go back behind the head on the same side they came up on, and tie the ends. Tuck in any gaps, and you're good to go. This works great for swimming - it's easy to find a scarf to match a swim suit, and you can pop a straw hat on your scarved head while you're lounging on the beach. A word of caution: you can get a sunburn through lightweight or light-colored scarves. Wear a sunscreen on your head, and wear a hat when you're not in the water.

Nothing accentuates a bald head more than a naked face. I'm talking about a face devoid of all hair: eyelashes and eyebrows. It's a dead giveaway. A wig can look as real as any head of hair could look, but if you have no facial hair, you might as well be wearing a chicken on your head for all the naturalness it would have. It's hard to believe you have a healthy, beautiful, full head of hair, when you can't even grow a decent eyebrow or two. So what can you do? Let me tell you!

## MAKEUP!

One woman I interviewed who had been through chemo

stated that without her facial hair, her makeup made her look like a clown. That's easy to imagine since there seems to be no definite outlines for your makeup to go into. It would be pretty frightening to get done putting on your makeup and have someone confuse you with that lady on the Drew Carey show.

After several years without hair, I have become quite proficient at applying makeup and making it look relatively natural. One tip I've found to be invaluable in eyebrow and eyeliner color is to pick a color that is *not* the same color as your hair. Look at several people and take note of their facial hair in comparison to the hair on their head. Most people's facial hair is darker than the hair on their head. I used a shade or two darker eyebrow pencil than my natural color for my eyebrows and eyeliner. This looks quite natural. As a matter of fact, I worked closely with another girl in a local hardware store for two years and it wasn't until I told her I had no facial hair that she noticed it was makeup.

I don't apply it too heavily, sometimes dabbing it with a tissue afterward to soften it a bit, or dust it lightly with translucent powder to make it last longer and not "melt" so quickly. When you follow the natural hair line of your eyebrows or eyelashes, you can't go wrong. You must be careful to start the eyebrow directly above the inside corner of the eye, and make short, wispy strokes (like hair), and end slightly past the outside corner of your eye. Create a natural arch just like your real eyebrows. I've even heard of a woman who makes a stencil to pencil in her brows to make sure they match. I do occasionally have difficulty making my brows exactly the same. Sometimes I find one eyebrow up a little higher, doing that critical, skeptical, "You're on the verge of trouble" thing that my mom always did with one eyebrow. I used to HATE that. I now do it to my kids. (Someone help me! I'm becoming my mother!!!)

Without makeup, your face can virtually disappear. It's important to wear your makeup the same way you did when you had hair. Eye shadow can look almost comical if there is no outline for it, such as penciled-in eyeliner or eyebrows. And when applying color to your face, remember: Natural. Less is more. If you've tried to apply your makeup and seem to be having trouble making it look like "you," you may want to go to a beauty salon that specializes in makeup and ask for help or advice. Ask them to teach you how to apply it. And most importantly, apply makeup in a well-lit area! A couple years ago, I was going to a basketball game with my husband, two of our children and another couple. Being of the "I'm not late, I'm just running a bit behind" gender, I applied my makeup in the van by the light of the visor mirror. When we got inside, one of my kids said, "Mom, why are your eyes red?" Suddenly, the crowd I was with burst into laughter. All they could manage to spit out was, "You'd better go check your makeup!" So I did. I got into the ladies' room, looked into the mirror and scared myself. It took me a moment to realize what had happened. I had mixed my rose lip liner pencil and my gray-brown eyeliner pencil. Gray-brown lips and red eyes. So, lighting, lighting, lighting!!!

There are some companies that specialize in hair replacement and false eyelashes and eyebrows that glue on, and you could probably find them in the yellow pages, most likely in the bigger cities. I have found false eyelashes in common department stores in the cosmetics section, but after putting them on, I thought I bore a striking resemblance to Tammy Faye, and gave them to my kids for Halloween. Besides, my real eyelashes never reached the middle of my forehead. Everyone would know they weren't "mine."

The most radical and daring type of cosmetics today is micropigmentation or blepharopigmentation. They're just fancy names for permanent makeup. Tatooing, if you will. It is done much the same as tattooing, but it's not as deeply introduced into the skin as the type of tattoo that you would see on any given Sailor. It has become much more common recently, and many of the major cities in the U.S. have at least one salon that does this or knows of one that can. If you have trouble locating a business that does this, you may want to contact the Department of Commerce for that particular state and ask them if they have record of any licensed beautician or plastic surgeon that does this procedure. You can also check with a local college of cosmetology. As with any costly and permanent surgical procedure, you must not hesitate, or be embarrassed, to ask many questions, such as:

1. Are you licensed?
2. Do you have references I can contact?
3. How long have you been doing this, and how many of these procedures have you done?
4. Are you insured?

5. Exactly what does this procedure entail?
6. How much does it cost, and how long will it last?

This procedure is considered permanent, but it does fade slightly after a few weeks, giving a softer, more natural appearance. It will continue to fade through the years, and you may eventually choose to repeat it.

Ask whatever and however many questions you can think of. This can be somewhat painful, physically and financially, and you need to be prepared. And don't make any decisions impulsively.

As a person with little or no hair, you may feel like you are trapped into a lifestyle or situation that you don't want to be in, and that you are up against a wall, with no choices or information to help you through this tough time. But you have many options. Your first decision should ultimately be to figure out what would make you happy, what would get you moving, what would force you to get on with your life. Do something, even if it's wrong, it's something. Nothing ventured is nothing gained, and all that. As I said earlier, you need to realize that you are worth whatever investment you make in yourself.

Chapter Nine

# Seeking Insurance Coverage for Cranial Prostheses

Getting insurance companies to cover full cranial prostheses.

First, check your policy for benefits and covered expenses. If it does not specifically exclude prosthesis, prosthetic devices, or treatments, you may be in luck. File a claim, including a doctor's letter or prescription stating the need for a hair prosthesis or treatment, a receipt for your hair prosthesis, signed by the provider (also have them sign your claim form), pictures of you without hair or makeup, and a personal account of the physical as well as psychological trauma and challenges associated with your hair loss. Also explain the costs of treatments and frequent wig purchases.

You should be prepared for denial of your claim. As I mentioned, if your policy does not specifically exclude prostheses, this may be your loophole. The challenge lies in convincing them that your hair is not just for cosmetic purposes. Your insurance carrier may simply deny your claim by stating that it is "not a covered benefit." The burden of proof is theirs. Get copies of your policy and list of your rights as the insured, and ask for an appeal. Ask for a review by a medical review board. You may need to explain the difference between a wig and a prosthesis, and the basic functions of body hair (see the forward in this book). Ask for a written reply. Insurance companies hesitate to put anything in writing that may be considered as "bad faith" in a future court case. When you send in your appeal, address it to a claims supervisor. You may end up getting the same claims person who denied it the first time, sure to deny it again. If all else fails, you may take them to small claims court. The most important factor in this step is: BE PREPARED!!! Have all correspondence records, letters, receipts, and names of every person involved in your claim process. Be sure to be able to account for all correspondence with dates, times, and full names and titles of everyone involved. You can even contact your State Insurance Commissioner to file a claim against your insurance company.

Legislation differs for each state as far as mandated coverage. You can work with your state legislature to adopt laws requiring insurance carriers to cover prostheses, including hair prostheses, and medical treatments that can aid you in regrowing your hair. The NAAF has very detailed information on how to convince your insurance carrier to cover the cost of a hair prosthesis or medical treatment. Feel free to contact them for this and any other information regarding hair loss and its challenges at this address:

The National Alopecia Areata Foundation
14 Mitchell Boulevard
San Rafael, CA 94903
Ph. 415-472-3780
Info@naaf.org

Chapter Ten

# "Hair"

*A Cowsills song devoted to, you got it, Hair.*

She asked him why
Why I'm a hairy guy
I'm hairy noon and nighty-night night
My hair is a fright
I'm hairy high and low
But don't ask me why
'Cause he don't know
It's not for lack of bread
Like the Grateful Dead
Darlin'

Gimme a head with hair
Long beautiful hair
Shinin', gleamin'
Streamin', flaxen, waxen

Give me down to there, hair
Shoulder length or longer, hair
Here, baby, there, mama
Everywhere, daddy, daddy

Hair, hair, hair, hair, hair, hair
Grow it, show it
Long as I can grow it
My hair

I can let it fly in the breeze
And get caught in the trees
Give a home for the fleas in my hair
A home for the fleas
A hive for the buzzin' bees
A nest for birds
There ain't no words
For the beauty, the splendor, the wonder
Of my

Hair, hair, hair, hair, hair, hair
Grow it, show it
Long as I can grow it
My hair

I want it long, straight, curly, fuzzy
Snaggy, shaggy, ratty, matsy
Oily, greasy, fleecy
Shinin', steamin', gleamin'
Flaxen, waxen
Knotted, polka-dotted
Twisted, beaded, braided
Powdered, flowered, and confettied
Mangled, tangled, spangled
And spaghettied!

Oh, say can you see
My eyes if you can
Then my hair's too short

Down to here
Down to there
Down to there
Down to where
It stops by itself
Don't never have to cut it
'Cause it stops by itself

Oh, gimme a head with hair
Long beautiful hair
Shinin', gleamin'
Streamin', flaxen, waxen

And won't you give me down to there, hair
Shoulder length or longer, hair
Here, baby, there, mama
Everywhere, daddy, daddy

Hair, hair, hair, hair, hair, hair
Grow it, show it
Long as I can grow it
My hair

Grow it, show it
Long as I can grow it
My hair

Hair.....[1]

## Big Hairy Deal
## or
## The Great "Love-of-Hair"

Hair sells. Never has a romance novel been written that doesn't include a detailed description of her lavish locks, "....and her lustrous, auburn tresses tumbled down her shoulders and over her heaving bosom like a cool, dark waterfall in the moonlight." Puh-lease.

Hair is a great love affair. We live in a society that worships hair, pays homage to it every day, and pays dearly. The expenses of hair related products and services alone are staggering. We're talking *BILLIONS\*!!*

Articles are written about hair: the do's and don't's, the newest trends, the latest fads, the care and treatments, the hassles and solutions, the best and the worst in Hollywood and across America. And, yes, some of these articles even report on the lack of it, calling it "Freakish," and "Bizarre,"

About 1/2 of the T. V. commercials on any given

---

[1] © Alfred Publishing. Reprinted with permission.

day are promoting hair care products. Shampoo, cream rinses, hair color, conditioning treatments, hair sprays, hair gels, hair freezes, foaming hair mousses, home perms, salon perms, shampoos that help curl your hair, perms that condition your hair, hair colors for permed hair, hair colors that condition, shampoos that color your hair, shampoos that simulate orgasms, (do they let minors buy that brand?), shampoos for dandruff and other unsightly conditions, shampoos that help grow hair, aaaaahhhh! After a while the ads become "white noise" like political ads. In one ear, out the other. And do you think that all this fuss is over HAIR! Nay, I say! It's about image! It's about vanity. It's about feeling good about how you look. That's not a bad thing. Society's obsession with looks is what's not healthy. Consider beauty pageants, for instance.

All the while we're talking about society's obsession with looks, how wrong it is, how we're truly enlightened, we're also feeling insecure, jealous, outcast, isolated, spurned, angry, bitter, and sad that we can't be "one of the beautiful people." Well, I've got a news flash for you. We are beautiful people. We're alive, aren't we? We're unique, interesting, creative, and resilient, right? It simply adds to our beauty to be hopeful, relatively happy, and loving. Think of one of the most beautiful people you know. How would you describe him or her? Are looks at the top of your list? I think of my Gramma Beulah. Was she physically attractive? Not particularly. I have beautiful thoughts of her, recalling her exact appearance, despite the fact that she's been gone for more than 35 years. At 67, she still had naturally black hair, only slightly peppered with gray, and always pulled back in a headband or goofy ponytail high on the back of her head. (Isn't it odd that hair should be the first characteristic I describe?) She always wore polyester slacks, a baggy sweatshirt with a safety pin attached to the front and a tissue stuffed up one sleeve. "You just never know when you'll need one of these things, Kissy." (- her knickname for me.) She was "plumpish," her bosom like a great glacier that slowly shifted southward over the decades. She was huggable, funny, generous, creative, and loving. Most of all, she was a constant in her grandchildren's lives, never too busy to visit, offer hugs, or dish up cottage cheese and peaches, her signature comfort food. She was a beautiful person. My point is that I can call to mind several beautiful people I know or have known and physical beauty has little to do with their qualifications as a beautiful person. So I'm constantly wondering why we can't be as kind to ourselves.

Hair plays a significant role in first impressions. In a recent magazine help column that I read, a woman was worried about what her future date would think of her because she was 30 pounds heavier than what she had previously told him. She was told that men usually first notice the face, hair, and eyes of a woman. I was immediately concerned. What if you don't have hair? Where does that leave you? Will he then ignore the bald head and move onto the eyes? Doubtful. Hair is simply the frame, but the face is the picture. Without hair, your face may as well be a blank canvas. So you had better draw fast, complete the picture, if you will, and make your face a landscape that rivals no other, complete with color, depth, and life. Or put something on your head if you're concerned about first impressions. Unless you're like me and depend on "The First Impression" to get rid of the life insurance salesman on your front step. Even after living without hair for years, I find myself making assumptions of and wondering about people who have no hair, although it is a *broader* range of assumptions. Perhaps he or she is going through chemotherapy, perhaps he has male pattern baldness in a *big* way, or perhaps he or she has alopecia. (Technically, anyone who suffers hair loss of any kind has alopecia. Remember, it is just Greek for "bald.") (Love those Greeks... they can make anything sound mysterious, classy...) Along with my impressions of these people come the overwhelming "Need to Know" feelings. I want to know all about them: who are they, why are they bald, what do they feel, what do they know, who do they know, what have they seen, found, read, experienced, felt, ...(Oprah syndrome.) Far more than anyone would want to share in the Target parking lot. But I have approached people, people who feel approachable, and I have been approached. And I must say that I am so glad that I appear to be approachable, and that others have felt comfortable approaching me about my baldness. It puts me at ease, and it makes me feel as though I'm helping others, if in no other way than satisfying their curiosity. And above all else, I feel that I have been successful in the impression I have given others. That I am comfortable with myself, and also with others.

As a matter of fact, I have even been comfortable enough to jog "topless," (but only in my neighborhood.) Strangers are the only ones who stare. I can only smile imagining what they must be thinking; "Poor dear .... got cancer and *still* she jogs! Bless her heart!" And sometimes I'm *so* comfortable with myself, my baldness, I forget why people may be staring at me, and wonder if I've dripped mustard on myself. That's ok. I'd probably look, too. Baldness isn't seen much. But it's also not that uncommon, only because of Alopecians' reluctance to bare all. I even considered running in a marathon, but after considering what people would assume of a bald woman running a marathon, I decided not to. (That, and the 26.2 miles……)

There are over two million people in this country who are bald because of alopecia. There are countless millions of people who have lost their hair, or are losing their hair, due to chemotherapy treatments, hereditary baldness, accidental baldness, and androgenic alopecia (male and female pattern baldness). To these millions of people, hair is a big deal.

There is little doubt as to the importance of hair. Minoxidil is proof of that fact. Rogaine, the brand name for Minoxidil, is a multi-million dollar seller. Its major consumer: men, condition: male pattern baldness. Minoxidil does sell to women, also, and a percentage of these consumers suffer from alopecia, but the intended goal of the company that markets Minoxidil targets men with pattern baldness.

*Cosmopolitan* magazine is a smart, savvy magazine with many wonderful qualities. But perhaps it should be called the *Body and Hair* magazine. It focuses so much on image and sexuality and trends that it sometimes fails to point out the importance of inner beauty and health. Rare is the issue that doesn't contain at least one article singularly focused on hair: the styles, the lengths, the problems, the care, the fads. This is not altogether bad, but tends to put too much emphasis on hair rather than the person who wears it.

Entire issues of certain magazines have been devoted solely to hair: *TV Guide*, for instance, with two Big Hair issues, one in December of 1995, and the next, their "second annual" Big Hair Issue, in April, 1997. (One of the articles was even called, "The Good, the Bald, and The Ugly.") The articles discussed the styles and trends in hair in Hollywood. Nothing new. Nothing profoundly fascinating. Just lots of talk of tresses. It's hard to dispute the importance of hair when one sees so many, many articles about hair. I've found them in *Family Circle, Readers Digest, TV Guide, Sun, Cosmo*, just to name a few. Not to mention hundreds of newspaper articles on hair and hair loss. So all you Alopecians/masochists, if you're looking for new and interesting ways to torture yourselves, look these up. Or simply turn on your television for 10 minutes.

Perhaps I'm more "hair aware" now that I have none, but is this "thing" with hair getting bigger all the time? Maybe the hype began with Farrah Fawcett's trendsetting hair style in the TV show, *Charlie's Angels*, which was a hit in the mid 70's. If you didn't have "Farrah hair," you were nowhere. Before "Farrah hair," long, straight hair was *soooo* in, that I know girls who actually ironed their hair. But once Farrah arrived on the scene, America's "babe wannabe's" dropped the steam iron and picked up the curling iron. (I *suspect* Farrah's popularity had little to do with her acting abilities.) Farrah is not alone in her trendsetting ways; there are several others who are known for their distinctive hair or hair styles, such as Cher, Tina Turner, Don King, Jennifer Aniston, Crystal Gale, Whoopi Goldberg, Dolly Parton, Dennis Rodman (bad as he wants to be and worse!), Alfalfa, Rapunzel, and Lady Godiva, to mention a few, and some who are known for their lack of it, such as Telly Savales *(major* crush!), Montel Williams, Yul Brenner, Mr. Clean, When you think of it, those who shave their heads are just *bald*-wannabe's. (I'm the *real thing!)*

There was a lot of hype when Demi shaved her head for a movie role. Then there was a lot of hype when it grew back. Bruce Willis shaved his head for a movie role. Hype. I don't recall who did it first, but they seemed to be competing for attention. Sinead O'Connor shaved her head for political reasons. Hype. Perhaps it's hype because they are taking a bold move in a world that worships what they chose to get rid of, if even for a short time.

Granted, it looks strange, but why does it need to be a big deal? Some brave, independent kids today are shaving their heads to be different. Almost all NBA players shave their heads. (I suppose it's because they can't afford hair care products.) It's a fad. But it will never be a long time trend and it will never be so common place that people wouldn't look twice at a bald head. Hair will always prevail, because it's safe, it's natural, and it's practical. And those of us who don't have it will more than likely choose the safe road of hair, fake or not, even if it's not the easiest road, just because we want to belong. Because we want to be just another hairy head in the crowd. Because if we wanted to look this way, we would have shaved our heads long ago when rebellion was in, and we would never have noticed that it didn't come back.

Some elite women of ancient Egypt shaved their heads and waxed and buffed them to a high sheen. Also in those days, entire Egyptian families shaved their heads and eyebrows in mourning when their cat died. (Bear in mind, their cats were also embalmed and had cemeteries of their own!) I tell you this so you know just how important cats were, not how unimportant hair was. As a matter of fact, ancient Egyptians had cures for thinning hair, such as lion's fat, a "guaranteed" cure.

Clayton Lehmann, a friend and Associate Professor of History at the University of South Dakota, mentioned to me once that he had found information about Alopecia Areata, or *alopekia,* in ancient Greek medical writings. Within this medical information was supposed causes and cures for baldness. Causes such as using the brain too much, (I should suffer from such a distinction!), slime, humidity deficiency, and "bad humors of the body." (Pardon me, but if it weren't for bad humor, I'd have no humor at all.) And Greeks and Egyptians had their own cures or treatments. Ancient Egyptian medical documents also include information about alopecia, like the papyrus found in 1873 in Luxor by the scholar Georg Ebers, appropriately named the Ebers papyrus, dating to the late sixteenth century BC. According to these documents, this is all you have to do to keep hair from falling out:

- Mix together ochre, collyrium, ht-plant, oil, gazelle dung, and hippopotamus fat, and rub the mixture on the head. (And I would do this right now .... if only *someone* knew what ht-plant was and where to get it!)
- Mix crushed flax seed with an equal quantity of oil, add water from a well, and rub the mixture on the head.
- Boil a lizard in oil and rub the oil on the head.
- Rub the head with castor oil and fat from a hippopotamus, a crocodile, a cat, a snake, and an ibex.

Other recommended treatments include dog's leg, donkey's hoof, fly droppings, dirt from under the fingernails, and hedgehog quills. Similar treatments were used to enhance hair growth or thicken the hair. (There's even a recipe to make a rival *lose* her hair.) Basically, their treatments aren't much different of those of today: inducing hair growth by contact dermatitis. In either case of ancient times of Egypt or Greece, one could proudly wear his or her bald head. Others would see you as someone who was really sad because your cat died, or you were thinking a lot. And I would much rather be bald and have these assumptions made of me than to carry around a towering hairstyle of such grand proportions, like that of Louis XV's times, that the doors at Versailles needed to be heightened to accommodate them. Imagine what the construction crew hired to do this work must have been thinking! (I'm sure it would look something like this: !!#^ ^/!!#%*@*%##*!#**!!!)

Society doesn't only worship hair, it perpetuates the prejudice against Alopecians by participating in the jokes and gags on them, as well. "Wigs coming off with the fish hook" and "Lady loses her hair" gags are categorized with "pants falling down" gags. I, myself, don't believe that it's wrong to have a sense of humor about whatever shortcomings we, as humans, have. I do believe that it's wrong to make fun of something that cannot be helped, or to be cruel to the point of laughing *at* someone, rather than *with* them. This is true of all people, whatever their condition or situation, not just people who lack hair.

But this chapter doesn't have to end there. True, we have no hair. There is no hype. We are bald without the fan fare. So not everyone knows. So we notice the second glances and curious children who are so blatantly innocent about staring. And the public will never be prepared to see bald heads, especially on women. So. What can we do? I'll tell you. We have two choices: Hide or get a life. I know what I'm going to do. And it doesn't matter whether others know I'm bald or not. The only way they will ever see me is how I let them see me, and I'm not talking about my head. Others will see me as a confident, fun, creative, interesting individual, with or without my hair, and I won't have it any other way. Maybe after they see me, they'll discover I don't have any hair. And it won't matter to them, either.

Chapter Eleven

# God Speaks

Spirituality and preserving our inner spirit.

Much of what I share with you in the next two chapters is just that: sharing. I have no experience in psychology or professional therapy unless you count being on the receiving end of it. (I believe I am a relatively well-balanced person, with the exception, of course, of my sense of humor.)

But of all the advice, professional help, and learning experiences I have had, I have to say that being able to relate to someone else in my situation, and the knowledge that I am not alone in my struggles with baldness, has been most helpful. So it is my hope that by relating (a lot), I may also help others deal with their hair loss.

This chapter deals both in spirituality and emotion. That's not to say you must be deeply religious or spiritual to be happy, but you should believe in yourself and your worth, if nothing else, in order to find peace, happiness, and fulfillment in your life.

It's human nature to question or blame the powers that be when something bad happens. That's not necessarily wrong, but what we do with our anger and our grief can have profound effects on both our spiritual and emotional foundations. And sometimes it is necessary, perhaps imperative, to re-evaluate our beliefs along with, and separate from, our feelings, so that therefore, we can nurture, cherish, and re-commit to them on a regular basis.

I believe that GOD SPEAKS to all of us. GOD SPEAKS to me through my dreams. GOD SPEAKS to me in church. GOD SPEAKS to me when I'm in the bathroom. (Honest! That's where I was the first time I ever "heard" Him.) Basically, GOD SPEAKS when I speak to Him. No, I don't hear God's voice. It may be something as subtle as an original thought. It may be a change in my mood, or a dream that shows me something in a different light. But regardless of what He says, when GOD SPEAKS, I listen. (I'm working on the "obey" part... )

Sometimes Satan speaks. And I plug my ears.

## SATAN SPEAKS

Oh, sweet insanity,
Oh, precious and everlasting death,
Save me from consciousness and suffering, And my
    constant awareness.
I am not strong.
I do not wish to be.
To Be.

Satan speaks.
Softly, sweetly.
He tickles my weaknesses.
He feeds my insecurities.
He dangles my peace in front of me. He smiles,
And waits patiently for me.
For Me.

cw

This poem is an expression of my depression. It puts a face on my emotion: Satan's face. I believe in God, therefore, I believe in Satan. I won't go so far as to say that Satan causes depression, but I'm sure he's got a slimy hand in it.

If your hair loss is affecting how you look at life, how you view the world around you, and how you think, and feel, and react, and *live,* then you may need professional counseling. I'm not ashamed to admit that I was deeply depressed and that I sought help. Allowing crappy feelings to control you is a habit; a habit more addicting and much more dangerous than biting nails or even smoking cigarettes. Depression is a habit. I'm not saying that to minimize it or make it sound trite or simplistic. It took a while for me to recognize my tendency to allow depression to hold me down. It was and still is, to some extent, easy to slide into a groove and let the bleakness guide me and my way of thinking, of perceiving the world around me. It's easy to lay down and die. It was easy to convince myself that everything was hopeless. I used to say, "It doesn't take much to convince me that life sucks." (I made that up!) I can't even tell you honestly that this attitude is *completely* past-tense.

I truly feel that one is never cured of depression. To be cured, in my opinion, is to have no trace of the illness left. But true depression is so deeply embedded in one's persona that it would be impossible, if not undesirable, to be completely rid of it. I feel one needs to remember, if even just a little, how he or she felt in order to help themselves, and perhaps others, enjoy life. "In remission" might better describe one's break from depression.

There are times when I'm not certain God is there. Maybe what I'm not certain of is my worthiness. But that is my insecurity talking to my head. I can honestly say that part of my problem with God is my anger. "OK., God. You did this to me. I hope you can live with yourself. But what's your point? Are you punishing me? Do you have some *greater plan* in mind? Maybe I don't want any part of it. Just give me back my hair. I'll be good."

When we don't have a logical explanation for what's happening to us, we assume it must be God's doing. Maybe I'm hoping that by giving God the cold shoulder He'll work some miracle on me to reaffirm my faith. It works on *"Touched by an Angel."* It's okay to be angry with God. Anger is a natural part of any real relationship, and just to say I have a relationship with God is comforting. Because even though I sometimes neglect Him, and try to pretend He's not there, or doesn't care, I feel He's a lifeline, a knotted rope hanging down in the dark, deep despair that I sometimes find myself in, bumping me, brushing against me, reminding me that

He's waiting, ready for me to grab hold if I get in too deep. But I really believe I am over the hump, and I will probably never be in too deep. I know He'll be there whenever I need Him.

In any case, by admitting my belief in God, I am admitting my belief in Satan. I truly believe, I must believe, that Satan wants me. By giving his face to my emotions, it is a little easier to resist destructive thoughts and impulses. This is what works for me. I haven't reached the point of "giving it to God." I'm still pouting. But I talk to God about other things. I avoid the subject of hair altogether. (I'm like a grounded teenager who wants to go to a dance. Do I ask? Do I try to earn my way back into favor? Or do I accept my challenge gracefully?)

This was an ongoing argument in my head. "Am I being punished? No. Maybe. I don't think so. What could I have done to warrant this? Nothing. I think." Sound familiar? That's what the old God did. This is the new and improved God. (Of course you know how Jesus changed all that, but to each his own belief.) Whatever your belief, you must maintain that you are not being punished. The heavenly penal code doesn't work that way. I was sitting in church a while back, half listening to the pastor's sermon and she said that God had my life planned before I was ever born. I woke up. I looked up. I felt betrayed. "What?!" I thought. "You mean You *knew* this was going to happen? *Some plan!*" But after I got past the feeling of betrayal and anger, I realized that God didn't do this to me, and if He did allow it to happen, He knew I would be the person to make something good of it. (I chose to believe this, after getting to know Him better and knowing that this is just the kind of thing He would do.) I even felt a *little* honored that He could trust me this much. That He could kick me in the pants to get me going in my writing and perhaps help someone in the process. Regardless, I won't blame God for my hair loss, but if my hair should come back, I will thank Him endlessly for it.

A dear friend of mine, Marlene B., once said, "God answers all prayers. Sometimes He just says no." It just might be that God doesn't say, "no," but that He says, "not now," or that He's waiting for us to figure out exactly what we're praying for or what we're needing, despite what it is we're asking of Him. Because when you think about it, when we pray for hair, or whatever thing we think we want or need, is that what we *really* want, or is it happiness? Acceptance? Peace? "Only our hairdresser knows for sure."

I'm not sure why I haven't just gotten down on my knees and asked God for hair. Maybe I'm afraid He'll say no, and I won't have any more chances to grow hair. Maybe I'm being forced to carry through on God's plan. Maybe I feel that there is so much strife in the world and so many more important things that deserve my prayers before a silly thing like my hair. I was brought up believing that I should pray for others first, and God will do what is best for me. Sometimes I just feel embarrassed that I could even think about hair when others are dealing with life and death issues, and I find I'm shaming myself into shape. Not long ago, I had a conversation with my sister-in-law, Deb, who had just been diagnosed with diabetes. She said to me, "I was thinking about you yesterday, Chris. I was brushing my hair and started wondering whether I would rather have alopecia or diabetes." I asked her, "What did you come up with?" And she replied, "I wasn't sure." I immediately realized that, even knowing what being bald was like, if I had to choose between alopecia and diabetes, I would choose alopecia. I don't think she was trying to say that my hair loss was insignificant compared to her diabetes, or that I should feel ashamed of my sadness over something so seemingly petty as hair. I think she was saying that everyone has a situation. And each of us has to evaluate what situation we're in, and make the best of life in that situation. I did read, however, of one woman who has both diabetes and alopecia, and she states that alopecia is the most traumatic for her to deal with because of the psychological impact. Although it does not diminish or eliminate the pain of my disease, I am in a state of perpetual thankfulness that I am healthy in every other respect.

It's probably a pretty safe bet that many of you feel as though you've been let down in the miracle department. It's understandable and perfectly acceptable to feel angry and disappointed. It's also perfectly ok to tell God what you're feeling. (P.S. He already knows, but if it makes you feel any better to voice it, knock yourself out.) Talk to God. Ask anyone: Prayer works. Whether it works because you're giving up control, or because God is at work, it works. Some people set aside a special time to pray. Some people pray a little all day long. That would be me. I like to talk to God whenever

I feel so moved; to thank Him, mostly, but also to ask for help on a regular basis. (Plus, I can say I was talking to God if someone overhears me talking to myself.) Some people are relaxed about prayer, some people are very disciplined about it. Look at Mother Theresa. I've heard there were grooves worn into the floor where she knelt everyday to pray at the foot of her bed. That really made me think: Didn't the woman ever rearrange her furniture? Anyway, talk to God. Talk to your pastor. Talk to yourself. You may just be surprised at what you hear in response.

My hair loss is of my body. My depression is of my emotions. I can't control my hair loss. I can't even control my emotions. But it is important to separate the two. There is a strong sense of loss of control that goes along with a loss one experiences. We spend our whole life learning how to control our time, our finances, our families, our homes, our bodies, and then something happens to prove to us that control is nothing more than a delusion. Because we can try as we might to control our surroundings, ourselves, but essentially there is no way to control outside influences on our lives. And when a change occurs without our "permission," we are baffled, frustrated, and left standing with our palms up and our mouths hanging open. These are the times that I need to remember that change is inevitable, that nothing is certain on earth, and that I am powerless to control anything that is not inside my head. I can *maintain*, I can *oversee*, and I can try to control my *reactions* to the things that happen beyond my control. So when I say that I can't control my hair loss, or my emotions,

I am simply stating that I have accepted change. I have accepted that loss, and loss of control is a given in life. The toll I must pay to gain is to lose also. Therefore, I can only control how I react to emotions, not the emotions themselves.

Controlling my reactions to feelings is not a simple task. I can't always be sunshine and happiness. Sometimes I just feel crappy. I can't help but feel crappy, and if I've had a crappy day, I'm going to feel crappy, and so be it. But I refuse to let those crappy feelings suffocate me. I now know the difference between bad moods, sadness, and depression. I talk to myself often and tell myself, "You are not depressed. You are mad, crabby, tired, sad, but it will not last forever. This, too, shall pass." There are days when I need to cry, so I do. There are days when I am crabby. We're human. We feel. Goodness and kindness do not always prevail. "I don't always wake up grouchy. Sometimes I let him sleep." (I love that one.) Yeah, occasionally I'm grouchy. So what. I don't bite. My bark works quite well. Barking never hurt anyone. (Dogs can teach us a lot!) I tell the clan I need to take a bath. I tell them I need to read. I tell them I need to take a break. I tell them if they don't leave me alone for at least 30 minutes they'll be eating pork liver and Lima beans for breakfast, lunch, and supper for a month. I get an hour. (They hate raw liver.)

If you have lost your hair, or had any kind of loss, you are entitled to feel crappy. You are entitled to be angry. You have suffered a loss and you need to grieve. I joined a loss group for a while and thought, at first, "I don't belong here. Everyone here has lost a loved one, gone through divorce, lost a job, lost the ability to do something, lost part of themselves... well, maybe I do belong here." It was very helpful to realize that even though hair's primary function *seems* to be cosmetic, losing hair was still like losing part of oneself. And, as with any other loss, the grieving process was the same. Elizabeth Kubler Ross, who is renowned for her writings on grief and grieving, wrote about the five stages of grief:

1. Denial - "This *can't* be happening to me. I don't believe it."
2. Anger - "Why me?! This just isn't fair!"
3. Bargaining - "Please, God, anything but this. I promise...."
4. Depression - "I just can't take it anymore. I don't know what to do..."
5. Acceptance - "Life goes on. I can handle it. I'm ok."

I went through every one of those stages. It's not uncommon to backslide before you get to acceptance. Acceptance doesn't necessarily mean that you won't grieve anymore either. You can reserve the right to grieve whenever you feel like it, and it's possible to accept it even though you may never like it. Acceptance doesn't even mean you've given up hope of a cure or the dream of getting your hair back again. It's helpful just to know what the stages of grieving are. I know that it helped me to realize that I was going through a normal process, that I wasn't insane, that I wasn't overreacting, and that it would get easier. Even as I wrote this book, I found myself going back into the chapters I had considered finished, changing, adding, and deleting as my attitudes about life and my baldness changed.

It's possible, probable, that you'll be told it's only hair; get over it. You'll likely be told you're lucky it's nothing serious, if that *is* the case. (If only I had a hair for every time I heard THAT one.) I can't tell you how to respond to things you'd rather not hear. I CAN offer suggestions... ask them if they've ever lost their hair then drop it. You could simply say, "Yeah, I've heard that...." You could say very honestly, "You're absolutely right. I am very lucky. But losing my hair is still very painful." You could smile and say nothing, my usual since I'm not confrontational. (I just go out and spit on their car.)

As with any loss, such as a death of a loved one, loss of a limb or mobility, or the ability to function in a normal capacity whether physically or mentally, people will tell you they know how you feel. It's a common reaction to be angry and bitter and tell them that they don't know how you feel till they've been through it themselves. Actually, they are not trying to be cruel and insensitive, they're just trying to help you through a rough time by sympathizing with you. But then again, no one has the right to tell you how you should feel or behave. It's one thing to sympathize with you, and try to be supportive and understanding. It's quite another to be condescending, minimizing your loss by telling you it's no big deal, get over it, and be thankful it's nothing more serious.

We have friends who lost a young child due to a farm accident a few years ago. They were grateful for all the love and support they received from family and friends and wouldn't complain about any comforts offered them in the painful days and weeks to follow. But through conversation afterwards, they mentioned some of the comments that well-meaning loved ones offered them, such as "It's God's will..." or "I know how you feel." or "At least you have other children..."

Just as our friends were subject to some thoughtless and almost cruel statements, they knew, as we should, that these people who shared their "wisdom" probably knew nothing of the pain our friends felt, and it wasn't the time or the place to teach them what their mama should have taught them long ago: Tact. And to be perfectly honest, I know I've said some pretty stupid things when I was just trying to be helpful, or funny, or sympathetic. It's part of human nature to speak before thinking. Most people don't try to be stupid. It just happens. Unfortunately, it happens a lot.

We'll never be able to completely avoid the comments that can hurt us. We can certainly make the decision to not let it hurt by remembering that for the most part, people don't usually intend to hurt us.

The healthy plant is not as likely to be overcome with bugs; the weaker plants are. In the same way, with a healthy attitude about ourselves, we can overcome the bugs. We can't be defeated unless we allow it to happen. We can be defeated by giving up or giving in to despair.

People who choose to be bald pave the way for those of us who have no choice in the matter. And guess what, folks! The only difference between *them* and *us* is ATTITUDE! My daughter has a T-shirt that says, "Attitude is everything!" I bought it for her, thinking it was statement of individuality, something that would be "cool." I discovered that it applied to every aspect of every life. I believe that no matter what you do, your attitude is the determining factor in whether it will be a success (next chapter) Attitude can't work miracles, but it can work. Attitude is the difference between staying down or getting back up. I keep thinking back to a joke: How many psychiatrists does it take to change a light bulb. None. The light bulb has to *want* to change. If you want to feel better, you have to *decide* that you want to feel better, then begin to *work* on feeling better, whether you do it on your own, or with help. It takes commitment. It takes tenacity. It takes time. And, yes, sometimes it takes help. Just knowing that there is a whole network of people out there who want to help makes that decision a little bit easier. If you suffer from alopecia, or any type of hair loss that is hard to cope with, you can contact the NAAF. They have an endless supply of information about alopecia, treatments, conferences, support groups, and techniques to help you live with your baldness. They also publish personal stories from others about their experiences with baldness, and there is nothing in this world like the feeling you get when you know you're not alone - someone else out there is feeling the same things, experiencing the same things, and thinking the same things as you. It's instant kinship. The NAAF is also constantly in touch with doctors and scientists who are studying alopecia, and therefore can give you up to date reports on their progress.

There is no shame in seeking professional counseling for helping us through a rough spot in our lives. Talk with your family doctor if you're not sure where to turn. He or she can recommend someone who would best serve your particular needs. If you don't have a support group in your area for alopecia or cancer patients, you can always attend one in a nearby town, or you could even start one yourself. You can even tell your doctor, dermatologist, or oncologist that you would be interested in speaking with someone who is going through the same thing you are, and tell him that he can give your name and phone number to the other patients if they would be interested in talking, or starting a support group. Some people feel as though they're strongest when they need to be strong for others. Helping others helps us! Go figure! There are lots of ways you can help yourself by helping others:

- Talk to someone who's bald.
- Visit oncology units and talk to patients who have lost their hair.
  Bring hats. Share stories.
- Get involved in something that *doesn't* focus on your baldness, like fundraisers for your favorite charity, for instance.

You may just want to choose a support person for you to talk to, like a sister, mother, close friend, brother, etc. I've also found it very helpful to journal. And it's good for a lot of laughs later when you read all the goofy things you wrote when you were just blowing off steam. (My journal is definitely NOT the type that old romance movies are made of!)

Another trend in therapy is hypnotherapy. It's doubtful that anyone can make you believe you have hair through hypnosis, but it may relieve some anxiety about baldness. I wish someone could hypnotize me, take me back in time and help me recall things just so I could update my baby books!

You are a worthwhile person and you just may not be aware of how great you are. Sit down sometime, when no one else is around to dispute your findings, and list your attributes. When I was feeling "less than," my counselors told me to list my attributes, my positives. At first, it was hard to sit down and try to think of how great I was. It was too easy to list my flaws. My brain hurt just trying to like myself. But the more I thought about it, the more I realized that I was not one big success, I was a whole bunch of little successes rolled up into one. Like a big Ho-Ho, layer after layer of good stuff. All of my attributes, little and big, make me a worthwhile person. Everyone is a worthwhile person because everyone has attributes. We can't help our flaws, we are not perfect, we'll never be, and that's why we are not God. (Bummer.) I wouldn't want that job anyway ... people calling all hours of the day and night.....

When I list my attributes, I list simple things like, "I'm a good bargain hunter." or "I have nice teeth." or "I'm short." (Yes, that can be an attribute!) "I'm forgiving." (That was a big thing.) The longer my list got, the more I realized that I'm not so bad, and who I am has nothing to do with my hair. When I was struggling with depression, I felt that everyone would be better off without me. But yet, when I think about friends or relatives that have committed suicide, I can't help thinking "What a waste!" "Their kids, friends, and parents will miss them so much. Didn't they know how much they were needed?" I could never apply the same logic to myself. Until I got help. Counseling did not make me a better person. I was pretty great to begin with. Counseling gave me the strength to change, to change the way I see myself, to change the way I think, to change from the habit of being depressed to that of being in control of my attitude. Like I said, I cannot always control my emotions, but I can control what they do to me.

Changing anything in our lives is a matter of discipline. I liken everything to dieting. It's easy to be lazy and indulge yourself in destructive behavior, like eating junk food. (Have I mentioned that I like Ho-Ho's?) Breaking any bad habit, like overeating, or smoking, or biting your nails is so difficult because it's habit; you do it without even thinking. You need to be on your toes. You need to be conscious of every little thing you do, and catch yourself when you start to act without thinking. Put that Ho-Ho down! Throw that cigarette out! Get that finger out of your mouth! Stop thinking! (Yeah, Right!) Yes. Stop thinking "like that." Don't indulge in destructive thoughts. Stop yourself, tell yourself to think of something good, positive, pleasant, and then get on with what you were doing. At first, you will feel silly thinking that you can't really change the way your mind works, but after you've done "self - talk" a few times, you will notice that you are not sliding backward. You are changing your way of thinking. And you are breaking a bad habit. (See the next chapter to know more about self - talk)

You're probably wondering how this chapter went from God to depression and on to attitude. I feel they are closely related. No, you don't have to believe in (a) God to be happy. But we all have a spiritual side to us that we rarely explore, or at least explore for *us* and *our* well being, rather than for others in their expectations of us. Well, I say, let's go spelunking. Put on our hard hats with the little light on it, and crawl in to our souls and find out what's in there.

I like to visualize my soul/my spirit as a cave. I imagine that there is a hidden entrance, that when I finally find it, it's a tight squeeze; I don't want to let myself in, or I'm secretly hoping I'll give up. It's dark, sometimes smelly and cold, but after searching awhile, I enter a large chamber where I can stand up and stretch. A place where I can go and just be "me" there.

We all have a "Spirit Cave" and we owe it to ourselves to find it. There are sure to be treasures not yet discovered, and treasures that we, ourselves, have buried and forgotten. Sometimes we need a guide. A spiritual guide like God, or a counselor, or a mentor, or even our stronger and braver selves, to navigate.

Sadness, self - loathing, bad habits, anger, hurt, all of these things can heap up on top of us without our ever knowing when it became such a burden. We can choose to drop this load and get on with life. We can choose happiness.

However, if it seems as though life is too much work, and you just can't seem to find any enjoyment or fulfillment in life, you may be suffering from severe depression and you need professional help. Please do not hesitate to ask for help from your physician or pastor or even a person you trust and with whom you feel comfortable. Life is short and very precious. Don't waste one more minute feeling miserable. True depression is not a "bad mood" or a "bad day," not imagined or simply "willed" away, but a clinical and treatable illness, sometimes caused by chemical imbalances, or attributed to a trauma or significant loss in one's life, or a combination of any of these.

Get help. Feel better.

I know that this is basic psychology, and I'm not a trained professional, I just know what works for me and that there is no bad advice in telling you to think better of yourself. Hair does not a person make. And I am qualified to tell you how you can live a full life without hair if only in the respect that I have no hair, and I am living a full and happy life.

Life *is* good.

Chapter Twelve
# It's All in Your Head
Attitude: Thinking, then acting.

B efore I begin this chapter, let me just say that I don't mean your hair is all inside your head. That is, unless you are an old man. From what I've heard, old men don't lose their hair; it just goes in and comes out somewhere else: the ears, the nose

When I begin to get overwhelmed with the prospect of living the rest of my life without hair, I just tell myself, "I don't have to live tomorrow yet. I can handle today. Today I'm ok." Self-talk. We all practice self-talk. Unfortunately, the self-talk we usually listen to is the negative type. "I can't. This is hopeless. Why bother." Well, it's all in your head. Your success in anything you do in life depends almost completely on your attitude. And where else is attitude but all in your head.

Motivation isn't about vitamins and caffeine. It's about *thinking* about what needs to be done. Dieting isn't about eating and food. It's about *thinking* about what you eat. Attitude about anything is directly affected by what you tell yourself. Attitude *is* what you tell yourself. If you say you can't, you won't. But if you say you can, you will. Because perseverance is an attitude. Tenacity is an attitude. Determination is an attitude. Ambition is an attitude. And good feelings are an attitude. Like Henry Ford said, "Whether you think you can or you can't, you're right."

Attitude is not something you can "get," it's something you have, and a gift you give yourself. You *can* change the way you think. By self-talk. Years ago I sold lingerie at home parties. And as everyone knows with home party sales, you are your own boss. And your own worst enemy. I was fortunate to have had a wonderful teacher and role model. A woman in New York named Carol McTiernan. She was very successful. (At everything she did!) And I know in my heart it was due largely to her attitude. She taught me to think differently. For instance, whenever I called her with a problem, she corrected me, and called it a "challenge." (To this day, I have a hard time saying the "P" word.) So if you consciously begin to adjust your self-talk from negative to positive, only good can come of it. And when I say, "Live today. Today I'm okay," and "One day at a time," I'm helping myself and changing the way I think, but more importantly, the way I feel. You can't be wussy about self-talk. You can't just mumble to yourself, saying things like, "I'm all right, I guess,... I think I might want to,... uh,... take, like, charge ... of my,... uh,... life..." No! You need to jump up onto your feet, and boldly tell yourself, out loud as well as loudly, "I deserve to be happy!" "I deserve to be good to myself!" "I am a great person!" Try it! It really works. And find a phrase or statement that works for you. Here are some suggestions:

"I feel good!"

"I like the way I look!"

"I like myself!"

"I am a fun and likable person!"

"I like my life!"

"I deserve to have fun!"

"I deserve to feel acceptable!"

"I deserve to enjoy my freedom from hair now and then!" (It's true!)

"I deserve to feel comfortable about my looks!"

"I'm good enough, I'm smart enough, and doggonit, people like me!" (oops, that's Stuart Smalley's line!)

These self-affirmations really work. The key to making them work for you, first of all, is to make them apply to you. You need to say them to yourself on a regular basis. Not just when you *do* feel good, but when you *need* to feel good. It may be necessary to say them to yourself several times a day at first. You may not even feel that what you're telling yourself is true at the time. Don't worry. You're not lying to yourself. You're convincing yourself that you are worthwhile. You are in a debate with the other part of yourself that would like to take the easy way out. Self-loathing is easy. Liking, *loving* yourself is work. But work with great rewards.

"One day at a time" was such an overused statement, that it held no meaning for me. That one phrase can turn me off and turn my stomach as much as the phrase, "Hold me .... Just hold me." (Don't you just HATE that line? It can spoil a whole movie for me. I've been known to never read another book by an author that uses that line in his or her book. They've lost all their credibility as a "good writer." It's as soap-opera-ish as cream of mushroom soup is Lutheran.)

Although, now that I've come up with my own personal adaptation of "One day at a time," ("I can handle today"), I can truly say it has saved me. From what, I don't know. Desperation, depression, anxiety, bitterness, and anger, probably. Maybe even death. I am honest enough to admit that I considered suicide. (Not because of my baldness or any other condition I was afflicted with besides depression, but baldness certainly didn't help.) I was **way** under. I didn't have a plan. I am incredibly disorganized. I just knew I wanted the pain to end. Continuous therapy implanted the quote in my mind, "Death is not an option." OK. So. What are my options?

1. Live.
2. See option #1.

There is only one way to live, and that is "for the moment." That's not to say that you shouldn't plan for tomorrow, or that you should act solely upon impulse. I have a plan. Often my husband will say to me, "What's the plan?" Meaning, "Do you have anything in mind for tonight?" And I always say, "I don't have a plan. That's the beauty of it all." Meaning, "I don't have a plan. That's the beauty of it all." (make it up as we go, be impulsive, don't have a plan...it's a beautiful thing.) But one time when I answered him this way, he said, "You've got to have a plan." It made me think. I still did not want every minute of every day planned out for me, but it did make me wonder what my goals are.

Goals are different from plans. Goals are necessary to enrich and challenge your life. Goals can be small, big, mediocre, anything as long as they are specific. And the goal is reached by having a plan. Thus, your first lesson in "Goal Setting - 101."

What are your goals? Do you have any goals for your career, your personal life, your hobbies? Getting out of bed every morning is one of my main goals. I love to sleep. It's my second favorite pastime. My first is none of your business. Therefore, I make it a goal of mine to tear myself away from this addiction. I promise myself an early bedtime, I promise myself a nap once a week, I promise myself just about anything to drag its lazy butt out of bed. Once I'm up and about I usually don't think about naps or sleeping until later in the evening. But I keep my promise of a nap if I feel I've earned it, or if I'm having a really crummy day and I desperately need it. (Like when I'm hormonal!) I've learned how closely connected the mind is to the body, and I know myself well enough now to respect my body's needs. When I'm beginning to feel overwhelmed and on the verge of whatever, I know I can contribute much of it to lack of rest. Sometimes I just know that a nap will help, even if I'm not lacking rest. (Ladies, blame PMS. It's a good way to allow yourself a crappy day once a month.) (Men, blame your wife's/sweetie's PMS. But not your wife/

sweetie!) I know I can't take care of anyone or anything else if I don't take care of myself first. It's not selfish if it's not excessive, it's just common sense.

Perhaps a good goal for you to have would be to be good to yourself. Treat yourself. (Not necessarily food. I've found that *backfires*.) Read a good book. Exercise. Buy a new wig or hat. Buy expensive shampoo and go home and lather up your head with it. *Nowhere* on the bottle of any of these luxurious, great smelling hair treatments does it specify exactly *how many* hairs you must have. There is no law prohibiting you from purchasing and using hair care products just because you have *no* hair, *a* hair, or *some* hairs. Someday I hope to have the nerve to go Au naturel' and purchase hair care products, just to see the reaction of the store clerk. Collect hats. Visit the museum. Whatever you do, pick something you really enjoy and commit to it. I treat myself everyday by taking the time to read while I have a cup of General Foods International Coffees' Suisse Mocha. One cup, every morning, no exceptions, for the last twenty years.

I'm still wondering what I'm going to be when I grow up. I'm only 50. Give me a small personal break. (I wanted to be Rosie O'Donnell, but that spot was taken.) Besides, life starts at 40. Actually, it takes all of my concentration and effort to raise four children and keep a household going, be it ever so bumpy. My day-to-day goals are usually written down on a list. Get out of bed, check. Make the bed, check. Get children off to school, check. Organize photo albums, ummmm, clean basement, uhhhh, laundry, half a check, everyday. My husband and I are both "list persons." The only difference between him and me is the number of realistic projects on the list and the number of checks at the end of the day. What really irks me is to complete a project, excited at the prospect of another check mark on my list, getting to the list, and discovering IT'S NOT ON THE LIST! OOOOHHHH! I then put it on the list and defiantly cross it off. It's my right as a "list person."

When you make your daily list, *if* you make a daily list, be sure to list your "want to's" as well as your "must do's." Do something good for yourself every day. If you're not a list person, write a love letter to yourself. (No need to get mushy and gross; just write yourself a letter saying what you'd like to do for yourself, what you want to do with your life, what would make you happy.) My "best" days are usually days that end with a feeling of accomplishment. Learning something I've always wanted to know or know how to do, getting to a project that I've been meaning to get to, or even simple things like having a clean house or creating a memory with one of my kids.

Above all, do what makes you feel good. (Within reason. Don't break any laws or hurt anyone!) Shopping is great fun, but it can be as addicting as chain smoking, and much more expensive. Something I learned is that "stuff" won't make me happy. (However, that doesn't stop me from testing this theory occasionally.) I can shop all day, have a marvelous time, then get home and ruin that good feeling thinking about the money I spent, even though I pride myself on being a bargain shopper, and usually stick to my shopping list. I realized awhile back that "stuff' is nothing if it doesn't mean anything to me. Most people don't keep family keepsakes and heirlooms because of their monetary value. It's worth so much because of the feeling they get when they see it. The memories it brings - the piece of Gramma that lives on.

I could sell some of the heirlooms I have for a few bucks, but the money would be gone, and more importantly, so would that feeling. And that good feeling is not about what looks good, but what feels good, even if it doesn't have the same effect on everyone else. I value the memories of my loved ones. I value the security and comfort of my memories. I value the feelings my loved ones have for me, and that, sometimes, is what sustains me when I'm feeling sorry for myself. I know that feeling good should come from within me, not from something I bought on impulse to fill a void. After all, feeling good is just that: a feeling. Sit down and write down some of your thoughts on what would make you feel good. Think of the things you enjoy doing. Maybe it's tennis, walking, quilting, reading, decorating, painting, gardening, volunteering, visiting, whatever it is, you are not being held back by your hair, or lack of it. Don't use your baldness as an excuse to let life pass you by.

I love to dance. I remember being so afraid to dance because my wig might fall off. I'm not a wild woman on the dance floor. What's the big deal? I've discovered that most people are understanding and compassionate and IF my hair fell off, I'd live through it, people around me would be polite, and the world would still keep spinning. Maybe those people would talk or laugh about it later, but I don't have to be there to hear it. And those people who would laugh out loud at the time, or make a cruel joke of it are not worth the embarrassment and shame and anguish that they would like me to feel. That doesn't mean it won't be painful, but I can know in my heart that I am a better person for living through it and not becoming bitter. The shame is theirs who cannot feel your embarrassment and pain. Later we will feel fine, and they will (hopefully) regret their behavior. In any case, their regrets are not our concern. I remember an incident with a friend of mine. He was telling us a joke and when he got to the punch line, his top teeth flew right out of his mouth onto the kitchen table! He laughed, we laughed (very hard, I must say) and his face was redder than the ripest tomato. However, he lived through it; we still love him dearly, and I wouldn't *dream* of telling *anyone* this story. (I mean, without his permission...)

One tip that might help you overcome your fear of "being discovered" is to wear a hat that covers your head but doesn't necessarily hide the fact that you have no hair. I've found that I'm not as concerned about a hat blowing off as much as a wig blowing off because I feel I've "prepared" people for the possibility or likelihood that I have no hair. So if my hat blows off, it should be no great surprise to them to see my bald head. A wig, as beautiful and "normal" as it makes me feel, also creates the image that I have hair and it certainly is more of a surprise to others when HAIR comes off. So if you're in a situation where your hair or hat could blow off, like at a park flying a kite, or at a balloon race, or on a sailboat, or water-skiing, or at the car wash with the top down, be prepared. Wear a hat. Or if you're comfortable with it, nothing at all. (You may want to wear some clothing. There are laws... ) Besides, the wax may be just the thing for a boring, dull scalp.

It would be nice if my first reflex to wind wouldn't be to grab my head, but it's at times like those when I'm thankful that I have reflexes at all. And fast ones, at that! Sometimes my reflexes are not quite fast enough. Like when we were leaving church one day, shortly after I began to wear a wig. It was slightly breezy, the norm for South Dakota, and when I opened the van door to get in, the wind rushed up behind me, swooped up and over the door, grabbing my hair, taunting me into a game of "Come and get it." It looked like some sort of hairy critter scuttling, rolling across the church parking lot. And more so than anywhere else in the world, I know "I am among friends." (Another quote I made up to cope with embarrassing situations.) But I immediately had visions of some women screaming and scrambling to their cars, children grabbing sticks to beat the "monster" with, and men, running, stomping, looking like they're trying to corral it like a spooked calf in their efforts to retrieve what they now know to be my wayward hair. "Melvin, it's coming your way! Grab it!" "It got away! Quick! Don! Go left! Left!" "There it goes!" I could see it all very clearly in my mind. Well, belying my panic and embarrassment, I simply asked Doug to go get it for me, which he did. I then threw it on the dash, and we drove home. Doug and I did manage to share a secret smile on our short drive home, but the kids were quiet, not knowing how mom was going to handle this. I'd rather they not assume too much, that everything embarrassing that happens, I want to laugh at, or just the opposite, I want to get angry or upset. I want them to learn to evaluate each situation to find out how the embarrassed person feels before they react. "Laugh with me, not at me." So they know I have to laugh first. (They know me well enough since I've lost my hair, that I'd much rather laugh. So we usually do.)

I hope, by now, that you have noticed that I have a sense of humor about my hairlessness. (Bizarre as my humor may be...) I make jokes about almost anything, and I have as far back as I can remember. I didn't gain a sense of humor when I lost my hair. It just gave me one more thing to joke about. I'll always choose a good comedy over a drama, or romance, unless they're really sappy or melodramatic, which instantly makes them a comedy to me. (Ever see the movie "*Wisdom*," directed by, produced by and starring Emilio Estevez? Watch closely in the "dramatic" helicopter scene with the special agents. One guy unintentionally does a great Chevy Chase impression. BIG laughs.) Stupid commercials and corny jokes are my favorite. "God only made a few perfect heads. And to the rest, He gave hair." "This is not a bald head. It's a solar panel for a love machine." "I'm not bald. I'm just taller than my hair." I also found a t-shirt that says, "I'm too sexy for my hair. That's why it isn't there." It goes good with my cap that says, "Another bad hair day, " and has a ponytail attached to the back.

Having a sense of humor has definitely given me strength, not just to deal with my hair loss, but to deal with other stresses in my life, children, housework, husbands, chaos, bills, breakdowns, just about anything. A sense of humor can be a very integral part of healing, both spiritually and physically. This is evidenced by Christine Clifford in her recent book *"Not Now .... I'm Having a No Hair Day"*, a wonderful book of humor and healing for people with cancer. Although Ms. Clifford's book does not focus solely on hair loss, as the title implies, she makes her point about hair loss being the most traumatic side effect of cancer treatment. Everyone knows there's nothing remotely funny about having cancer, but having humor about everyday occurrences, even those that happen to people with cancer, can make the gloomiest days a lot brighter. Laughter has a natural ability to ease tension. It's a well known fact that laughter releases endorphins, a necessary chemical in the brain that can ease pain, relax, promote healing, and lift the spirits.

One of the first times I laughed at my baldness was when my first husband asked me to pull the blind in our bedroom because the moonlight bouncing off my head was keeping him awake. I wasn't even completely bald. This condition was new and scary and still painful for me. But in spite of myself, I laughed. I guess I forgot it was painful for just a moment, and allowed my sense of humor to take over. Sometimes you have to laugh just to keep from crying, kind of like wiping out on your bike when the other kids are watching. The laughter comes, and then comes the healing. I suppose I've done my share of both laughing and crying, but it's the laughter that makes me feel better. As much as being bald hurts, it won't kill me. There were times that I wish I didn't have to live with this affliction, but not so much that I would choose to end my life. Admittedly, there are times that nothing can take the place of a good cry. Anyone who suffers a loss is entitled to that. Eventually, the pain lessens and it's much easier to handle the everyday calamities that come along.

In the original formation of this book, I saved a special section just for humor. After working on it for months, I figured out why that section was so empty. It's because happiness, or humor, isn't something you can force. You have to allow it to happen to you. You have to see it, create it, live it and let it come through in every part of your life. I couldn't write just about humor. I could only write about humorous things that happened to me in everyday occurrences. I could only laugh at things because of the way I perceived them. Maybe everyone wouldn't find the same things as humorous. Like one time, my sister, Brenda, and I took washable markers and drew hair on my head, complete with a braid going down my neck. Another time when I was with Brenda, we were playing with a huge batch of gak I had made (the stuff that looks like snot - and I *would* say "feels like," but who would admit to knowing *that* -, except this was pink) and had gotten out for the kids to play with. I love this stuff! I took my scarf off, slapped it on top of my head, and let it ooze down over my face while I recited the preamble to the constitution. It really was quite funny (to us), and the kids were in stitches.

(I suppose that was because I couldn't remember the last few words to the preamble.) My husband, whose sense of humor is as dry as my tuna casserole, (sorry, Doug.), just said to me, "You are weird." That's a fact. I am weird. But I love to be silly and I love to laugh and make people laugh. What's the harm in that? Laughter is good for everyone.

I used to be appalled when I would see someone laugh at a funeral reception. I got over that when I caught myself laughing at a funeral reception once. Humans see humor in spite of, and sometimes instead of, pain. We smile at a funny memory, we rejoice in togetherness, we are relieved when we find out this is not the end of the world. Of course things will never be the same. Things are always changing. But we cope, and a great part of coping is acceptance. And how could we accept ourselves and our situations without a certain amount of humor.

Shortly after I began dating Doug, we were shopping for a card for a wedding we were going to attend. And it was right around the time of my birthday, so he was also looking for a card for me. When you've only been dating a few weeks, you need to be careful not to get a card that's too serious, too cutesy, too mushy, too platonic, too personal. It's quite a challenge. I saw Doug smiling. I figured he had found just the card. But instead of purchasing it, he showed it to me. On the front it read:

*I can still see you standing on the hill,*
*your hair blowing in the wind*

and on the inside:

*And, you, too dignified to run after it.*

We cracked up laughing. Part of me was blushing, but part of me said, "GOOD ONE!"

I'll always regret not buying that card. (It wasn't a birthday card, but a "missing you" card. It just wasn't appropriate. And I guess I wouldn't know "appropriate" if it came up and kicked me in the pants.)

Part of the reason I try to see the funny side of things is to put others at ease. I know it's not my job to make everyone comfortable with my baldness. It's not their cross to bear. They can walk away with their hair. (Poem!) But I like people to know I'm not sensitive about it, either. I can be hurt as easily as anyone else in the face of cruelty, but I don't encounter much of that. Cruelty can only come from ignorance, and it's ignorance that warrants the pity. So when people find themselves talking about hair, or the perm they just got, or how they "just can't do a thing with this hair!" I chime right in and say, "I know what you mean. This hair right here just won't do what I want.... like SPREAD!" I pick up on their embarrassment when they catch themselves talking about hair, and immediately try to relieve it with humor. I feel so much better about myself knowing that I made an uncomfortable situation easier to deal with. Besides, I would much rather be known for my ability to cope, to laugh, to accept, to help, than for my tendencies toward self-pity or bitterness. That's not the person I want to be. I want to be known as someone who's organized, talented, tenacious, fun to be around, interesting, intelligent, (we can't have everything, now can we?), well, you get the picture. I may not excel in all these areas, but I like to challenge myself. When I find myself saying something like, "I can't do that...." I stop and ask myself, "Why not?" So, I learned basic plumbing. I learned how to do scherenschnitte (paper cutting). I learned how to re-upholster. I learned to paint roses. If I can learn all those things, surely, I can learn to live with a little ol' thing like baldness. Compared to all of the wonderful things and tragic things in life, baldness is a little thing.

It's a common assumption that bad things don't happen to celebrities. We conveniently forget to list people like Lou Gherig, Sharon Tate, Marilyn Monroe, Buddy Holly, Christopher Reeves, Gilda Radner, Erma Bombeck, and countless others among the tragedies. Yes, even celebrities go through the struggles us "regular" people go through. Point is, they are "regular" people. They just have "irregular" exposure. Princess Caroline has alopecia. Carol Channing has alopecia. Oprah Winfrey lost her hair once because of some hair treatment gone awry. Many people know that Humphry Bogart died of lung cancer, but the fact that he had alopecia is not so well known. It's also ironic that my favorite coffee cup has a picture of "Bogie" on it, with the quote, "Hair's lookin' at you, kid." I got it free with a perm at a local hair salon years ago. I wasn't even bald at the time. (Duh! What would I have permed, my ears?) Incidentally, I also have a cup from a dinner theatre we attended which reads, "Social Security." And, like "Hair," however entitled, needy, or deserving I may be, there's no guarantee I'll get that either!

So, I may go on hoping and praying for hair, or a cure, but I'm certainly not going to waste one minute waiting for it before getting on with my life. I can accept myself the way I am today, and if someday my hair comes back, or a cure is found, Hallelujah! Until then, I've got stuff to do.

Epilogue
# "A House of a Different Color"

You're renting a spacious, beautiful house that you've grown quite fond of over the years. The rent is cheap, the landlord is wonderful, you've fixed the place up *just* the way you like, you couldn't possibly be more comfortable or happy in any other home. Sadly, your landlord dies, his son is your new landlord, and he assures you he will be just as good a landlord as his father, if not better.

Well, things roll along fine. Then one day you return home from a week's vacation. Your new landlord is standing in front of your freshly painted house wiping his hands on a rag, and admiring the fine job that was completed just moments before your arrival.

Your house is now purple. A very brilliant purple. Shiny, Barney purple. With orange, yellow, and fuchsia trim. You want to cry. (Go ahead. I would. I'm glad *I* don't live there.) You're speechless. Your landlord, on the other hand, is literally quivering with excitement and pride. You smile/wince, quietly thank him, and comment that you are grateful that your house will be easy for your dates to find. You slip inside your front door, drop your bags, and bawl your head off.

Several boxes of tissue later, the shock has worn off. The redness has disappeared from your nose. You've gathered yourself, and begin to formulate a plan, everything short of moving, which is out of the question. You could "accidently" burn the house down. (No, you love this house. That would be a waste. All the things you care about are inside it.) You could pray for a tornado that might strip the house of all its paint. (Fat chance.) You could plant many trees around it and fertilize them hourly. (No, that would still take too long.) You could wear a disguise. (No, everyone already knows who you are and where you live.) You could offer to repaint the house at your expense. (No, you don't want to spend all that money painting a newly painted house.) You begin to accept it, and tell yourself, "It's only cosmetic. The inside, where I *really* live, is still the same. I don't have to look at it... much. It's the same house, the same safe, comfortable place I come home to, and the rent is still cheap. The landlord, aside from the fact that he's a color blind lunatic, is still nice, and he *is* kind of cute..." (You see where I'm going here?)

So, you continue life as you knew it, or something somewhat close to that. You patiently answer children's innocent questions, and constantly reassure them, "No, this is not where Barney lives." You tolerate the blatant stares, the occasional snickers, and rationalize that if they really knew who lived inside, the color of the house wouldn't really matter. You live on the inside, not seeing the outside like everyone else does. And from the inside looking out, everything is the same. You have the same likes and dislikes, the same talents, the same sense of humor, the same tastes, the same personality, the same fears and insecurities, and the same friends and family. You are still the same person. Only the outside of where you live is different. Not bad, not ugly, just different.

# The End

Living with baldness is the same as living with any other physical difference. We need to live from the inside out. We need to remember that what others see is not what is. What we see is not what is. Who we really are is what is. The word "flaw" should only apply to actions, not physical attributes. Sadly, this is not what is.

Isn't it ironic that only when we are old (and I'm not saying that I'm old) and have lived and learned life's lessons for ourselves that we can know how important it is to accept ourselves and others for who we are, and that we cannot impart this wisdom, via bribery nor jack hammer, to the young, impressionable, and eager.

b

As I get older, and my life does not seem to be waiting for me, I realize how important everyone is to me. Everyone I know, or know of, and even those who I don't care for, are important to me. They are important because of what they can teach me. They teach me what I should be, what I could be, what I like and don't like, and most of all, what I don't want to become. I have learned how to help myself, how to help others, how easy honesty is, how effortless despair can be, and how difficult it can be to ask for help. I only wish someone could have given me this advice: Get out of your own way.

I've been standing in my own way for half of my life. All of the obstacles I claim to have had were nothing more than excuses. I realize now that my goal in living with hair loss, or any other of life's challenges, is not to seek approval or acceptance from others, much less to try to impress them. It should be our goal to accept and love ourselves. Live our lives inside out. Ultimately, it is our duty to ourselves, our gift to ourselves, to determine, to decide, to celebrate the fact that we are no less whole, no *less*, than those with hair. We are merely different. Not one of us is the same as another. Thank God.

# Resources

Dr. Scott Ecklund, Family Practitioner, Sanford Family Medicine, Sioux Falls, SD

Dr. Gene Burrish, Dermatologist, Sanford Dermatology, Sioux Falls, SD

National Alopecia Areata Foundation newsletters

Journal of the American Academy of Dermatology

Magazine and newspaper articles:

Family Circle, April, 1983

Cosmopolitan, 1985

People, Sept., 1986

TV Guide, Dec., 1985, April, 1997

Readers Digest, Oct., 1985

Omaha World-Herald, Sept., 1981, Jan., 1983, June, 1986

www.ingramcontent.com/pod-product-compliance
Lightning Source LLC
LaVergne TN
LVHW010214070526
838199LV00062B/4580